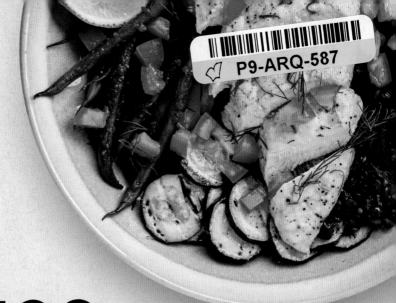

P9-ARQ-587

100
WEIGHT LOSS
BOWLS

Heather
Whinney

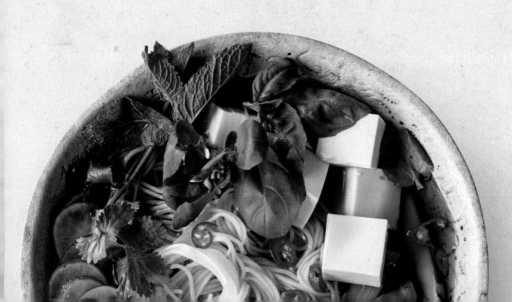

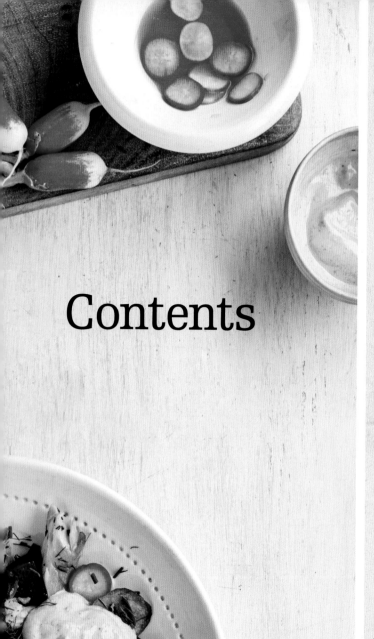

Contents

Smoked
mackerel hash
with harissa yogurt
(see p74)

Weekend brunch 54

No-cook bowls 80

Speedy bowls 118

Relaxed meals 152

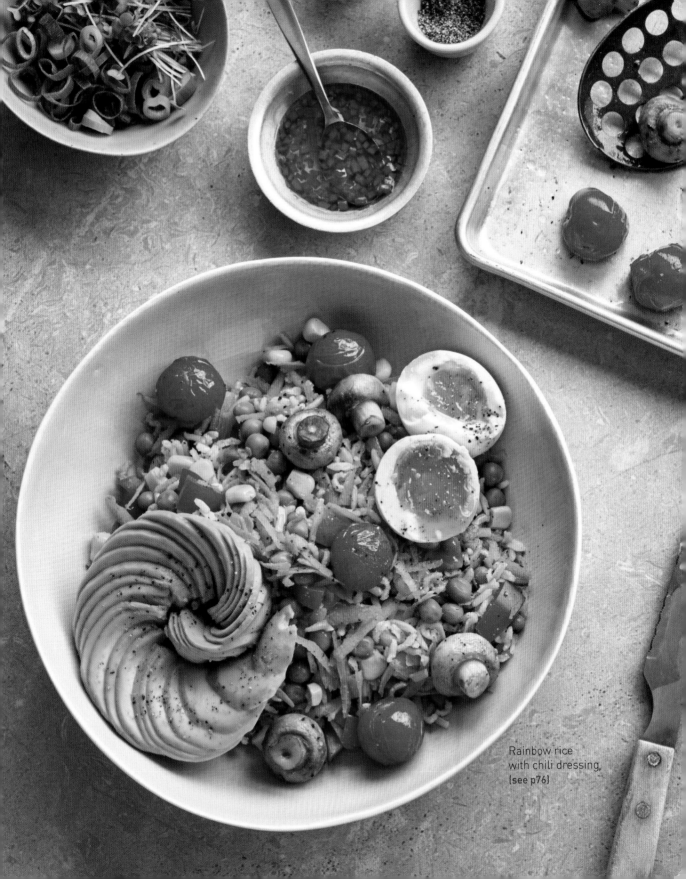

Rainbow rice
with chili dressing,
(see p76)

Ready, set, bowl!

Eating from a bowl is the simple way to enjoy delicious, complete meals while controlling the amount of calories you take in. And the great recipes and practical guidance in this book will help you reach your weight loss goal with ease. So let's get started!

Why eat from a bowl?

Life today feels increasingly busy, and it can be hard to keep track of your weight. So a quick-to-prepare one-bowl meal of colorful, tasty food hits the spot when you need a healthy energy boost that's comforting and filling, but low in calories.

Bowls are the new plates

Food from a bowl can help with portion control: a bowl can typically hold less food than a dinner plate, allowing you to monitor your portion sizes and keep them consistent, while still providing you with an ample meal. Because of their rounded shape, bowls give the illusion of greater volume compared to plates, tricking your brain into believing that food served from a bowl is more substantial than exactly the same amount presented on a plate.

Bowl recipes should have a balanced blend of gutsy flavors: sweet, sour, bitter, salty, and umami. And the broad range of herbs, spices, seeds, and dressings you can add increases their flavor without adding significant calories. Portability is also a bonus: because bowl food is designed to be a complete meal, it's the perfect on-the-go solution, so you won't have to resort to bad choices when out and about.

Enjoy your food

Certain foods are best served in a particular way, which explains why a meal can look more interesting and taste better when it's served in a bowl. When we eat, our senses are impacted by the look of food first, then its texture and flavor, which increases the amount of pleasure we take in eating, and even our perception of how satisfied and full we feel at the end.

A balanced meal

By choosing a balance of healthy food groups that combine together well in one dish—whole grains, lean protein, vegetables, and a sauce or dressing—you can control the ingredients you use and avoid hidden or unnecessary calories. This nutritionally complete approach will also help keep you feeling fuller for longer, so you won't need to snack: a bowl of creamy avocado, juicy tomatoes, tender fish, and crunchy greens, for example, works not only because of its nutritional content and appealing color, but also because it has a balance of textures that contributes to a feeling of being satiated.

> Bowl food is gaining popularity because it can increase the pleasure of meals.

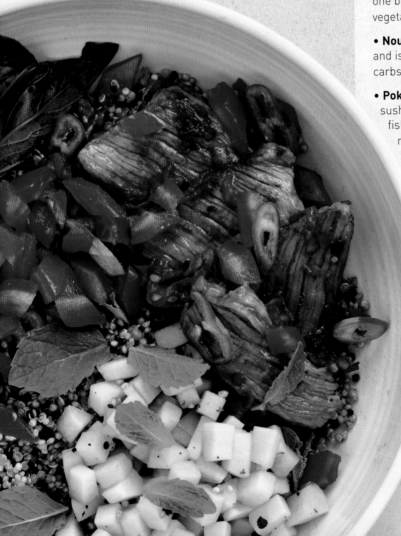

A bowl-based plan for the future

It's a simple formula, but it works well: a fiber-rich diet with lots of lean protein and vegetables in a bowl will help with gradual and sustained weight loss. It's also a fun, creative way to eat and is extremely versatile: you can very easily adapt the ingredients you use and how you prepare them according to the season, such as including raw ingredients for extra color and crunch in summer, or opting for a warming bowl of hot food in winter.

What's in a name?

You may hear different names for bowl foods, both within these pages and in restaurants, so here's a guide to the most common.

• **Acai:** Features the superfood acai berry, which provides antioxidants and a tangy taste that's ideal for bowl food

• **Breakfast:** Designed to keep you fuller for longer, these will often use eggs, pulses, or beans for protein

• **Buddha:** Looks like Buddha's belly: piled high with veggies, beans, nuts, and/or grains

• **Hippie:** Features multiple superfoods in one bowl, such as quinoa, seeds, berries, vegetables, and more

• **Nourish:** Looks like a salad in a bowl and is usually overflowing with protein, carbs, and healthy fats

• **Poke (poh-kay):** A bowl of deconstructed sushi, Hawaiian-style, this starts with raw fish and is commonly served with sushi rice and vegetables

• **Power:** A super-balanced bowl full of protein and power foods to give you all-day energy

• **Rice:** Starts with a base of rice (typically brown) and is topped with meat or fish and vegetables

• **Smoothie:** Blends fruits and/ or vegetables into a morning meal and is topped with nuts or seeds for a crunchy finish

• **Sushi:** Essentially a take on a sushi roll-in-a-bowl, combining healthy fats, sea vegetables, and sushi rice

What makes a nutritious
weight loss bowl?

Balanced, calorie-controlled meals are key to weight loss. Bowl food fits the bill perfectly if you choose good-quality ingredients from crucial food groups and follow a few simple guidelines.

Your nutritional needs

For optimum health and vitality, your body requires a range of essential nutrients every day. If you also want to lose weight, every bite must matter, so you don't have to consume unwanted extra calories. Start with the premise that most of your meal must consist of complex carbohydrates—such as whole grains and vegetables—which also provide much-needed fiber. Add smaller proportions of lean protein and beneficial fats and you have the basis for the ideal, nutritious weight loss bowl.

Complex carbohydrates

Fresh vegetables and whole grains are called complex carbohydrates because they contain plenty of fiber, which is slowly broken down by the body into a steady supply of glucose that fuels the body's cells and enables you to function at every level, from breathing to exercise. Refined foods, known as simple carbohydrates, contain no fiber and are quickly converted by the body into glucose, creating a swift energy surge that can soon leave you feeling tired and hungry again.

Make sure at least half the ingredients in your bowl are complex carbohydrates such as brown rice, oats, beans, legumes, and an array of fresh vegetables, which will maximize your intake of minerals, vitamins, fiber, and antioxidants.

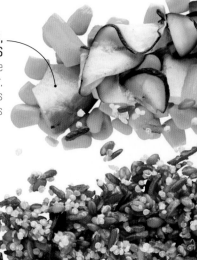

MEAT, FISH, AND TOFU
Provide **protein** and **fats**, but stick to lean cuts of meat to keep the saturated fat down

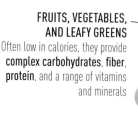

FRUITS, VEGETABLES, AND LEAFY GREENS
Often low in calories, they provide **complex carbohydrates, fiber, protein**, and a range of vitamins and minerals

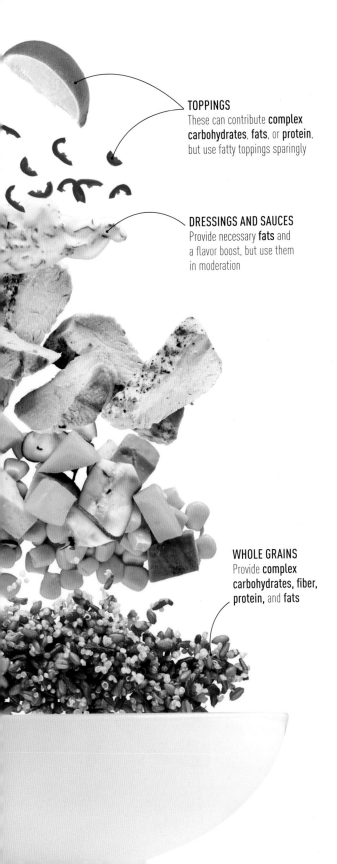

TOPPINGS
These can contribute **complex carbohydrates**, **fats**, or **protein**, but use fatty toppings sparingly

DRESSINGS AND SAUCES
Provide necessary **fats** and a flavor boost, but use them in moderation

WHOLE GRAINS
Provide **complex carbohydrates, fiber, protein,** and **fats**

Protein

The second crucial food group is lean protein. It takes the body longer to break down protein than carbohydrates, so eating protein ensures you'll have steadily regulated glucose levels over several hours and leaves you feeling fuller for longer. In addition, lean proteins—such as tofu, fish, eggs, and chicken—are known as "complete proteins" because they provide crucial amino acids that the body needs to function effectively. Make sure that approximately a quarter of your bowl is made up of lean protein.

Monounsaturated fat

The days when all fat was deemed bad if you were on a weight loss program are over; now you just need to choose your fats carefully. Monounsaturated, or essential, fats contained in such foods as avocados, olive oil, nuts, and seeds contain many beneficial nutrients that are also crucial for the body to work properly. These essential fats take even longer for the body to break down than carbohydrates or protein, further slowing the rate at which your food is converted into glucose and making them the third indispensable food group. It's the texture, or "mouthfeel," of these beneficial fats that can enhance your eating experience and help you feel full. However, you don't need huge amounts of essential fats; they should make up about 20 percent of a meal.

Saturated fat

There is a place for certain saturated fats in a weight loss plan: coconut oil, some cuts of meat, and dairy products in small amounts all provide the body with useful nutrients. However, if you find you crave fatty foods, try including monounsaturated fats—such as avocados and nuts—into your bowls, and you may find you no longer reach for nutrient-poor foods, such as donuts.

Target your
daily calorie intake

A well-balanced bowl is loaded with vitamins, minerals, and other essential nutrients, but it also contains calories, which are the measure of how much energy food contains. Tracking your calorie intake can help you meet your weight loss target.

How much weight will you lose?

Knowing how many calories you need to eat each day for weight loss is crucial to achieving your goal, and many factors— such as your age, height, metabolism, and activity level—can impact your daily caloric requirements. The weight loss calorie targets in this book are based on eating 500 fewer calories than the recommended daily intake from the USDA (see right). That adds up to a total of 3,500 fewer calories each week, or about 1lb (450g) of weight loss. So you will lose weight slowly and steadily by following this approach; your body will also benefit from the gradual process, easily adjusting to the changes in your daily calorie intake and steady weight loss.

When should you eat your calories?

Eating isn't an exact science, but following some basic guidelines can help ensure you're putting together a meal plan that spreads your calorie intake throughout the day. Try to regulate your meals and snacks so you don't go more than four hours during the day without eating. This method should help to prevent any dips in your glucose levels, which can cause energy crashes that make you reach for unhealthy snacks, sending you over your daily calorie target.

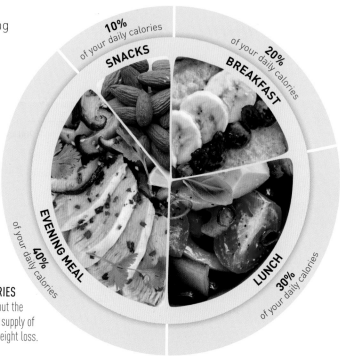

10% of your daily calories
SNACKS

20% of your daily calories
BREAKFAST

30% of your daily calories
LUNCH

40% of your daily calories
EVENING MEAL

DISTRIBUTE YOUR CALORIES
Spread your food throughout the day to give you a constant supply of energy and aid your weight loss.

Determining your daily calorie needs

The charts below offer guidelines for determining the number of calories you should consume each day in order to maintain or lose weight.

Begin by finding your activity level on the chart for your gender, then your age range.

The right-hand column shows the number of calories you should consume daily for healthy weight loss: 500 calories fewer than the recommended number of calories a day for weight maintenance. (If you want to lose weight more quickly, consult your doctor.)

Daily calorie intakes for men

AGE	SEDENTARY		MODERATELY ACTIVE		ACTIVE	
	RECOMMENDED CALORIES	CALORIES FOR WEIGHT LOSS	RECOMMENDED CALORIES	CALORIES FOR WEIGHT LOSS	RECOMMENDED CALORIES	CALORIES FOR WEIGHT LOSS
21–25	2,400	**1,900**	2,800	**2,300**	3,000	**2,500**
26–30	2,400	**1,900**	2,800	**2,300**	3,000	**2,500**
31–35	2,400	**1,900**	2,600	**2,100**	2,800	**2,300**
36–40	2,400	**1,900**	2,600	**2,100**	2,800	**2,300**
41–45	2,200	**1,700**	2,600	**2,100**	2,800	**2,300**
46–50	2,200	**1,700**	2,400	**1,900**	2,800	**2,300**
51–55	2,200	**1,700**	2,400	**1,900**	2,800	**2,300**
56–60	2,200	**1,700**	2,400	**1,900**	2,400	**1,900**
61–70	2,000	**1,500**	2,200	**1,700**	2,400	**1,900**

Daily calorie intakes for women

AGE	SEDENTARY		MODERATELY ACTIVE		ACTIVE	
	RECOMMENDED CALORIES	CALORIES FOR WEIGHT LOSS	RECOMMENDED CALORIES	CALORIES FOR WEIGHT LOSS	RECOMMENDED CALORIES	CALORIES FOR WEIGHT LOSS
21–25	2,000	**1,500**	2,200	**1,700**	2,400	**1,900**
26–30	1,800	**1,300**	2,000	**1,500**	2,400	**1,900**
31–35	1,800	**1,300**	2,000	**1,500**	2,200	**1,700**
36–40	1,800	**1,300**	2,000	**1,500**	2,200	**1,700**
41–45	1,800	**1,300**	2,000	**1,500**	2,200	**1,700**
46–50	1,600	**1,100**	2,000	**1,500**	2,200	**1,700**
51–55	1,600	**1,100**	1,800	**1,300**	2,200	**1,700**
56–60	1,600	**1,100**	1,800	**1,300**	2,200	**1,700**
61–70	1,600	**1,100**	1,800	**1,300**	2,000	**1,500**

Creating your **weight loss plan**

Now that you've determined your daily calorie needs for healthy weight loss, you can build a well-rounded, calorie-controlled meal plan of bowl foods and snacks.

How to create your meal plan

Each recipe in this book gives you the information you need to put together a daily, weekly, or monthly meal plan that fits with your calorie and dietary needs. Every recipe is clearly labeled as under 300, 400, or 600 calories, making it simple to identify and choose recipes for your tailored plan.

1 **Your daily calorie target**
Using the information and guidelines on the previous pages, determine your personal daily calorie intake needed for healthy weight loss (500 calories fewer than the daily recommended calories needed for weight maintenance).

How to plan a day

This sample meal plan uses a combination of bowls and snacks to meet your daily calorie needs and help you stay full. It's based on a daily weight loss calorie target of 1,500 calories, the requirements of a moderately active 26–50-year-old woman.

 UNDER 300 CALS Breakfast **+** **UNDER 100 CALS** Mid-morning snack **+** **UNDER 400 CALS** Lunch

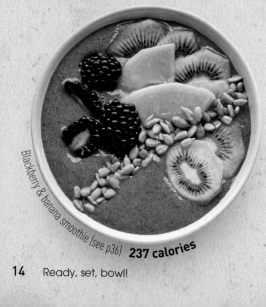
Blackberry & banana smoothie (see p36) **237 calories**

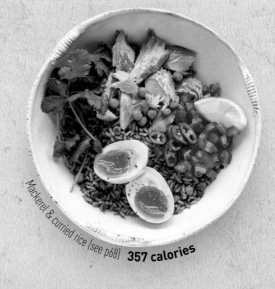
Mackerel & curried rice (see p68) **357 calories**

2 Pick your bowls

Choose three bowls with calorie counts that together add up to about 200 calories fewer than your daily calorie target. Each recipe and its nutrition information is based on a single serving, and bowls are categorized by meal, preparation speed, or portability, allowing you to make a meal plan that fits with your lifestyle.

3 Complement meals with snacks

Use snacks to bridge the calorie deficit between the three bowls and your daily calorie target (see below). Snacking between meals will keep you from feeling hungry and prevent low blood-glucose levels, which means you're unlikely to resort to unhealthy snacking or overeating at meal times.

UNDER 100 CALS Smart snacking

Below are examples of snacks with fewer than 100 calories. Add two to your three-bowls-a-day meal plan to help you meet your goals and keep you feeling full between meals.

- 1 pear, 1 orange, or a small banana
- 12oz (350g) chopped watermelon
- 5oz (140g) 0% fat Greek yogurt, 1 tsp honey, and a little ground cinnamon
- 1 rice cake with 2 tsp almond butter
- 14 whole almonds
- 12 baby carrots with 2 tbsp hummus

- 10 baked tortilla chips with 4 tbsp salsa (any heat)
- 4½oz (125g) blueberries with 1 tbsp flaked almonds
- 1 medjool date filled with 1 tsp almond butter
- 4½oz (125g) berries

Icons for special diets

On each recipe you'll find icons that indicate if the recipe is compatible with a dairy-free, gluten-free, or vegan diet.

DF = Dairy free   **GF** = Gluten free   **VG** = Vegan

+ UNDER **100** CALS Afternoon snack + UNDER **600** CALS Dinner = About 1,377 calories

You're under your calorie goal for the day!

Turkey & mango (see p132) **583 calories**

Remember the impact that calories in drinks can have on weight loss. Don't forget to factor them into your calorie goal.

Supporting your
weight loss plan

Changing your eating habits isn't the only thing you can do to help you lose weight. Becoming more active, eliminating calorie and sugar traps from your diet, and tracking your progress will also help you meet your weight loss goal.

Include exercise

Just as with healthy eating choices, the key to establishing exercise habits that easily become a part of your daily routine is to start slowly and be consistent. You don't need to set yourself big fitness goals from day one; even small, simple changes such as taking the stairs instead of the elevator or going for an evening stroll can help to burn more calories than usual, and so help to reduce your weight.

Refuel and reevaluate

When you eat after exercising, choose something with lean protein or complex carbohydrates to help your muscles recover. Try to eat within 30 minutes to two hours after exercising, as that's when your body will be looking to refuel and repair itself.

If you change your exercise habits drastically, remember to reevaluate your daily calorie target for weight loss and adjust your meal plans accordingly.

How many calories can I burn in 30 minutes?

Not all exercise is created equal when it comes to burning calories. The more intense the exercise, and the more muscles you use, the more calories you will burn. This illustration represents the number of calories typically burned by performing 30 minutes of each of these common forms of exercise.

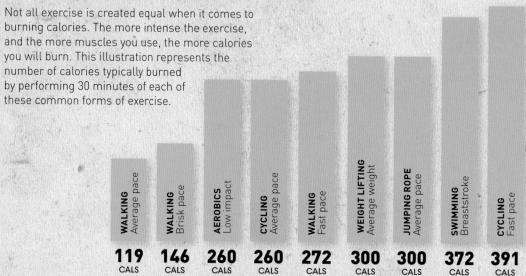

WALKING Average pace	WALKING Brisk pace	AEROBICS Low impact	CYCLING Average pace	WALKING Fast pace	WEIGHT LIFTING Average weight	JUMPING ROPE Average pace	SWIMMING Breaststroke	CYCLING Fast pace
119 CALS	**146** CALS	**260** CALS	**260** CALS	**272** CALS	**300** CALS	**300** CALS	**372** CALS	**391** CALS

Avoid sugar traps

The World Health Organization recommends keeping your daily sugar intake at less than six teaspoons, but most of us consume far more than that. Many seemingly healthy foods contain hidden sugars, making them high in calories and likely to cause swings in your blood-glucose levels. A teaspoon (4g) of sugar provides you with 16 calories.

It's important to always read food labels. A few common sugar traps are ready-made granolas, some of which have as much sugar per serving as a chocolate peanut-butter cup; store-bought sauces, dressings, and dips, with one tablespoon of ketchup often containing almost one teaspoon of sugar; and fruit juices, with some containing just as much—or even more—sugar than there is in a can of cola.

Track your progress

Tracking your weight loss, exercise, and food choices can be very motivating, while also holding you accountable. Having to write down that cookie you ate might make you think twice about eating it in the first place!

There are numerous websites and apps you can use to help track your progress, many of which are free. Most will help you monitor your weight and track your goals, what you eat, and how much you exercise. Some will also give you daily reports on your progress.

Even writing down by hand what you eat and how much exercise you do might help you to see where you're going wrong, and determine any changes you need to make.

No matter which option you choose, be honest with your recording.

Drink smart

You need about eight 8fl oz (240ml) cups of liquid a day to stay hydrated and ensure your body is functioning properly, and even more if you're exercising. However, some drinks can be full of hidden calories and sugar, which will quickly derail your weight loss. Below are some suggestions for smart choices... and for options it's best to avoid.

Drink

✓ Water

✓ Hot water with lemon

✓ Herbal teas

✓ Fruit teas

✓ Occasional no- or low-sugar tea and coffee

✓ Matcha green tea

Avoid

✗ Sugary drinks, such as soda, energy drinks, or sweetened iced tea

✗ Too much sugar added to tea or coffee

✗ Sugary fruit juices

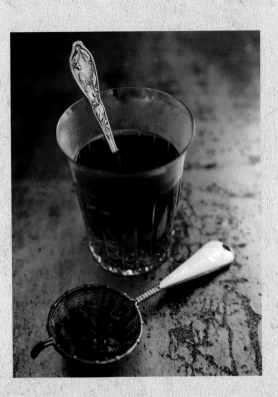

FLAVOR WITHOUT CALORIES
Herbal and fruit teas are refreshing and full of flavor, so you can skip the soda.

Planning and prepping

Once you've worked out your meal plan, it's easy to create a shopping list to go with it. Having all the ingredients on hand and as many items as possible prepared in advance will help ensure you reach for healthy options instead of instant junk food.

Shop ahead

For many people, the easiest way to prepare in advance is to focus on the week ahead. Start by creating your meal plan for the week. You can save time during the week by choosing recipes with similar key ingredients so you can batch-cook and have them ready to use when it's time to assemble your bowl. Once you have your meal plan, make a shopping list of everything you'll need. It's important to stick to your list when out shopping; if there's no junk food in the house, then there's none available to eat when you get hungry.

Prep ahead

At the same time that you make your shopping list for the week, read through the recipes to see if there's anything you can cook in batches to cut down on prep time during the week, and make a note of it. Most foods can be cooked in advance, safely stored in the fridge, and used within four days, but check food safety guidelines if in doubt. Your freezer can also be very useful when it comes to prep. Many foods can be frozen (see right), so you can cook more than you need and then save portions for when you're ready to use them in the future.

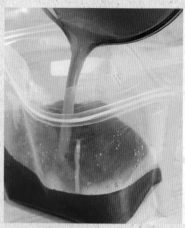
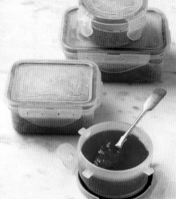

PORTION OUT EXTRAS
For convenience, store extras in single-portion airtight containers or bags. Refrigerate or freeze leftovers as soon as they're cool. Never leave them out for longer than two hours.

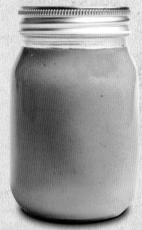

SMOOTHIES
Properly stored, a smoothie can be kept in the freezer for up to three months.

Fruits and vegetables

• Because cut produce spoils relatively quickly, try to prep fruits and vegetables just before use. Precut produce will keep for two days in the fridge, so, if you must prep produce in advance, make sure to use sealed containers or bags. Cover vegetables with cold water before refrigerating.

• Treat fruits and vegetables with lemon juice or wrap them tightly in plastic wrap to minimize oxidation when storing them.

• Don't wash any fruits or vegetables until you're ready to use them; the extra moisture can cause spoilage.

Grains

• Cooked rice can be kept in an airtight container in the fridge and safely eaten within 24 hours, but be sure to reheat it thoroughly. You can try to plan your meals so you cook two portions of rice together and then use a portion in your bowl one evening and the other as part of your lunch or dinner the next day.

• Cooked grains, including rice, can be stored in the freezer for up to one month. If you can cook a big batch and freeze it in individual portions, it can be a great time-saver. If you do plan to do this, it's better to cook the grains until they're al dente, so, when reheated, they won't be overcooked. Always thoroughly reheat them once they've defrosted.

Smoothies

• Make smoothies in advance by blending ingredients as directed, then keeping them in the fridge for two to four days, depending on the ingredients.

• You can freeze smoothies for up to three months.

Dressings

• Prepare dressings for the week ahead. Keep them in glass jars in the fridge, shaking the jars before each use.

• Dressings will keep for up to one week in the fridge, but they don't usually freeze well. Only make what you need for the week, to reduce waste.

Marinades

• If you have time, marinate any meat or fish the night before you plan to use it. This gives the ingredients time to properly absorb into the meat and intensifies the flavor.

• While it might be tempting, never reuse marinades that have come into contact with meat. This can spread germs and cause food poisoning. Discard any leftover marinade immediately after using.

What can you freeze?

Preparing and freezing ingredients in advance will save time when it comes to making bowls. While most things can be frozen, some are better fresh because their texture can change or they can break down once defrosted. Here is a guide to foods that do and don't freeze well.

Freezes well

✓ Avocados (mashed)
✓ Bananas (sliced and peeled)
✓ Berries (freeze on a tray first to prevent sticking together)
✓ Chili peppers
✓ Cooked rice and grains
✓ Dairy or almond milk
✓ Garlic (peeled)
✓ Ginger (peeled)
✓ Herbs (can't be used for garnish once defrosted)
✓ Hummus
✓ Lemongrass
✓ Lemon and lime (cut into pieces)
✓ Meat (cooked or uncooked, in portions)
✓ Pesto (in portions)
✓ Raw eggs (shell removed)
✓ Silken or firm tofu

Doesn't freeze well

✗ Cooked fish
✗ Soft cheeses with a high water content
✗ Watery vegetables and fruits, such as lettuce, cucumbers, bean sprouts, radishes, or watermelon
✗ Yogurt

Bowl boosters

When added to the bowls in this book, these power foods will turbo-charge a meal's nutritional value and its flavors without having a big impact on the calorie count.

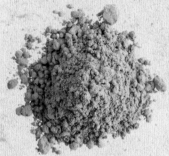

MATCHA
Matcha—a type of powdered green tea—has been found to contain 20 times more antioxidants than there are in either blueberries or pomegranates.

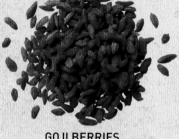

GOJI BERRIES
(go-jee)
Goji berries have been used for centuries in herbal medicine. They contain vitamins C, B_{12}, and A; iron; selenium; and other antioxidants.

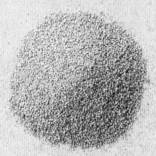

QUINOA
(keen-wah)
Quinoa is gluten-free and is one of only a few plant foods that are considered a complete protein, containing all nine essential amino acids.

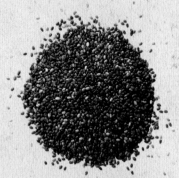

CHIA SEEDS
Chia seeds grow to about 10 times their size in liquid, expanding in your stomach and making you feel full. They're 40 percent fiber by weight and also contain more omega-3s, gram for gram, than salmon.

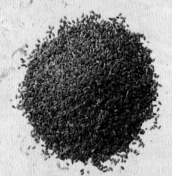

FLAXSEEDS
These seeds are gluten-free and high in antioxidants, fiber, and omega-3 fatty acids. They also contain lignans, which might provide some protection against cancers that are sensitive to hormones.

ACAI
(ah-SIGH-ee)
Acai berries contain amino acids, fiber, essential fatty acids, vitamins, and minerals. Some studies have shown they have more antioxidants than raspberries, blackberries, or strawberries.

> Antioxidants are thought to protect against the harmful effects of free radicals, which are known to cause cell damage.

Super seed toppers

Using seeds as a topping is a quick and easy way to boost flavor and nutrition. Most seeds are good sources of fiber, minerals, and essential fats.

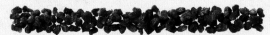

POMEGRANATE
Loaded with fiber and vitamin C, and good for your heart

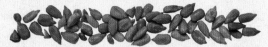

SUNFLOWER
Chewy and nutty, with inflammation-fighting vitamin E as well as selenium

SESAME
Nutty and helpful in fighting high blood pressure and diabetes

NIGELLA
Slightly peppery, with cancer-fighting compounds such as thymoquinone

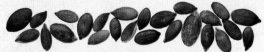

PUMPKIN
Mildly nutty, with magnesium and immune-boosting zinc

POPPY
Slightly fruity and full of phosphorus and calcium for strong bones and teeth

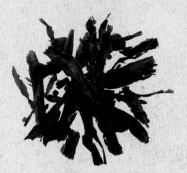

SEA VEGETABLES
Sea vegetables—or edible seaweeds—are low in calories and provide fiber, iodine, and lignans. Many studies have shown that they're also a potent source of antioxidants.

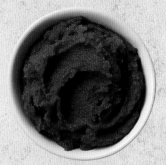

MISO
Miso is made from fermented soybeans that are turned into a paste. Fermented foods are good for digestion, and miso contains all the essential amino acids and is high in B vitamins and antioxidants.

Bonus recipes

Store-bought sauces, dips, and dressings contain too many hidden calories for use in a weight loss program. Making your own means you have full control over exactly what goes into them—and you can count the calories per serving.

Edamame & wasabi dip

makes ABOUT 1¼ CUPS / 5 SERVINGS   prep 5 MIN   cook NONE   serving size ¼ cup

Want to add a little spice to a bowl? This dip offers a rush of heat tempered by creamy, cooling yogurt.

Calories **99**	Cholesterol **0mg**	Dietary fiber **2.5g**
Total fat **4g**	Sodium **1mg**	Sugars **0.2g**
Saturated fat **0.5g**	Carbohydrates **0mg**	Protein **8g**

the INGREDIENTS

115g (4oz) frozen edamame beans (soybeans)

½–1 tsp wasabi, to taste

2 garlic cloves, peeled and roughly chopped

1 tbsp 0% fat plain Greek yogurt

handful fresh mint leaves

sea salt and freshly ground black pepper

the PREP

1 Put the edamame in a bowl and cover them with boiling water. Leave for 3–4 minutes, then drain.

2 Put the edamame, wasabi, garlic, yogurt, and mint in a food processor, season with salt and pepper, and process until well combined, adding 4 tablespoons of hot water. Taste, then add more wasabi or seasoning as needed.

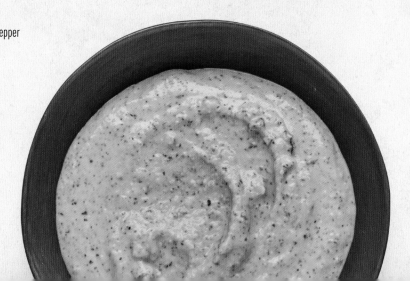

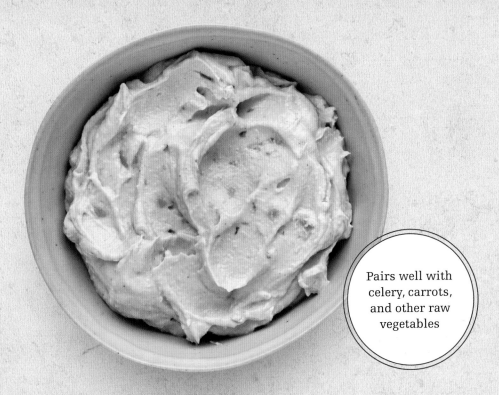

Pairs well with celery, carrots, and other raw vegetables

Oil-free hummus

makes 1½ cups / 5 SERVINGS   prep 5 MIN   cook NONE   serving size ¼ cup

Enjoy this Middle Eastern classic without worrying about adding too many calories to your snacks.

Calories **68**	Cholesterol **0mg**	Dietary fiber **3g**
Total fat **2.5g**	Sodium **0.1mg**	Sugars **0.2g**
Saturated fat **0.5g**	Carbohydrates **7g**	Protein **3.5g**

the INGREDIENTS

3 cups chickpeas, drained

juice of 1 lemon

1 tbsp tahini

pinch of zatar (optional)

sea salt and freshly ground black pepper

the PREP

1   Put the chickpeas in a food processor and process until ground but still chunky.

2   Add the lemon juice, tahini, and zatar (if using), then season with salt and pepper to taste, and process again until well combined. With the food processor running, add ½ cup of hot water until the mixture becomes smooth, or more if you'd like it smoother. Taste, then add more seasoning and blend again if desired.

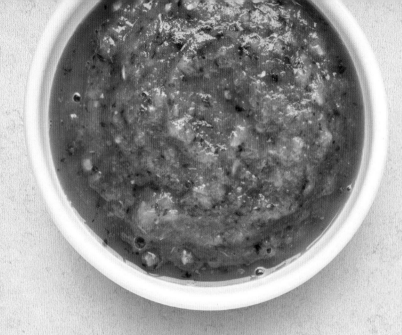

Roasted tomato *salsa*

makes **2 CUPS / 8 SERVINGS**   prep **10 MIN**   cook **20 MIN**   serving size **¼ CUP**

This delicious salsa is something you can make ahead and keep in a sealed jar in your fridge, ready for use anytime.

Calories **9**	Cholesterol **0mg**	Dietary fiber **0.5g**
Total fat **0.2g**	Sodium **1mg**	Sugars **1g**
Saturated fat **0g**	Carbohydrates **1g**	Protein **0.3g**

the INGREDIENTS

6 tomatoes, halved

1–2 red chili peppers, to taste

4 garlic cloves

1 tsp olive oil

sea salt and freshly ground black pepper

1 small red onion, finely chopped

handful of cilantro leaves

juice of 1 lime, plus extra if needed

the PREP

1 Preheat the oven to 400°F (200°C) and mix the tomatoes, chili peppers, garlic, and olive oil in a roasting pan, seasoning with salt and pepper. Roast for 20 minutes or until the tomatoes and peppers begin to blacken.

2 Blend the roasted garlic and chili peppers in a food processor until well chopped. Add the tomatoes, red onion, cilantro, and some more salt and pepper to the food processor and pulse-blend. Add the lime juice and pulse again until the salsa is at your desired consistency. (It should retain some texture.) Taste, then add more seasoning or lime juice as needed.

Sriracha sauce

makes 1 CUP / 8 SERVINGS   prep 5 MIN   cook 10 MIN   serving size ⅛ CUP

This can turn any bowl into a spicy meal with great nutritional value, but without adding many calories.

Calories **13**	Cholesterol **0mg**	Dietary fiber **0.5g**
Total fat **0g**	Sodium **2mg**	Sugars **2.5g**
Saturated fat **0g**	Carbohydrates **2.5g**	Protein **0.5g**

the INGREDIENTS

½ cup red chili pepper, roughly chopped

1 romano red pepper, seeds removed, roughly chopped

3 garlic cloves

1 tbsp apple cider vinegar

1 tsp tomato purée

1 tsp honey

sea salt and freshly ground black pepper

the PREP

1 Put the chilis, romano pepper, garlic, apple cider vinegar, tomato purée, and honey in a food processor, then season with salt and pepper. Add ½ cup of hot water and process until blended.

2 Pour the mixture into a small saucepan and bring to a boil, then reduce the heat to a gentle simmer and cook for 10 minutes. Taste the sauce, then add more seasoning as needed.

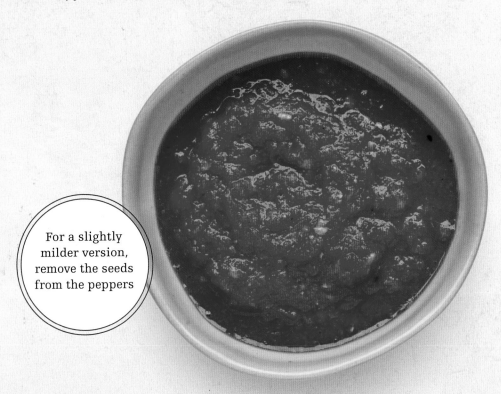

For a slightly milder version, remove the seeds from the peppers

Skinny ranch dressing

makes 2½ CUPS / 20 SERVINGS   prep **10 MIN**   cook **NONE**   serving size ⅛ CUP

You don't have to sacrifice flavor when trying to lose weight. This dressing is an ideal addition to any salad bowl.

Calories **54**	Cholesterol **0mg**	Dietary fiber **3g**
Total fat **2.5g**	Sodium **2mg**	Sugars **5g**
Saturated fat **0.5g**	Carbohydrates **5g**	Protein **1.5g**

the INGREDIENTS

2 tbsp silken tofu

1 tbsp apple cider vinegar

2 tsp Dijon mustard

sea salt and freshly ground black pepper

8½oz (240g) low-fat buttermilk

1 tsp finely chopped dill

1 tsp finely chopped flat-leaf parsley

1 tsp finely chopped chives

the PREP

1 Blend the silken tofu, apple cider vinegar, and Dijon mustard in a food processor, then season with salt and pepper before blending again.

2 Add the buttermilk, dill, flat-leaf parsley, and chives to the food processor and blend until smooth. Taste the dressing, then adjust the seasoning as needed. (Refrigerate the remaining servings for up to 2 weeks.)

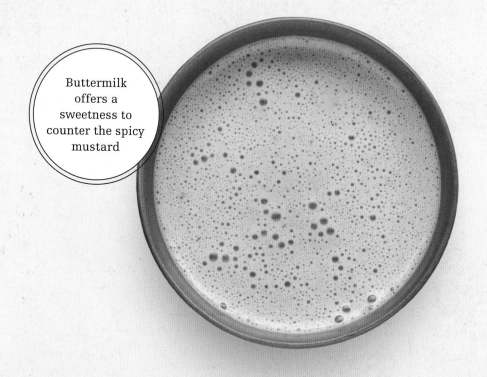

Buttermilk offers a sweetness to counter the spicy mustard

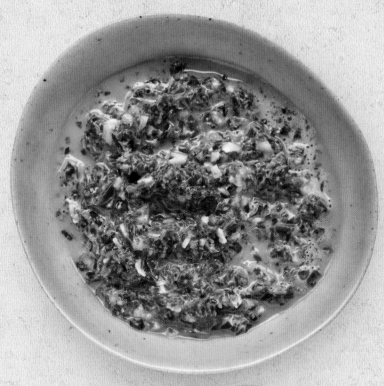

Kale pesto

makes **2 CUPS / 8 SERVINGS**   prep **5 MIN**   cook **NONE**   serving size ¼ **CUP**

Soothing kale and fiery red pepper flakes add Mediterranean zing that will enhance almost any bowl in this book.

Calories **77**	Cholesterol **0mg**	Dietary fiber **2g**
Total fat **6.5g**	Sodium **22mg**	Sugars **0.8g**
Saturated fat **0.7g**	Carbohydrates **1g**	Protein **3g**

the INGREDIENTS

5¾oz (160g) kale, coarse stalks removed, leaves roughly chopped

large handful of basil leaves

3 garlic cloves

1 tbsp extra virgin olive oil

pinch of red pepper flakes, or to taste

¼ cup almond flakes

sea salt and freshly ground black pepper

the PREP

1 Blend the kale in a food processer until well broken down, then add the basil leaves and process again.

2 Add the garlic, extra virgin olive oil, and red pepper flakes and process again until well combined.

3 Add the almond flakes, season with salt and pepper and process once again. Taste the pesto, then add more seasoning or red pepper flakes as needed. Loosen the consistency with 1–2 tbsp of water, if you like.

Quick-start breakfasts

Breakfast provides essential energy to kick-start both your metabolism and your day. These bowls all contain exciting flavors that will help boost your weight loss.

Oat & quinoa porridge
with cinnamon & banana

prep **5 MIN**   cook **20 MIN**

Adding cinnamon to this creamy, hearty porridge gives a spicy kick to the soothing oats and quinoa.

Calories **348**	Cholesterol **0mg**	Dietary fiber **5g**
Total fat **7g**	Sodium **182mg**	Sugars **30g**
Saturated fat **0.8g**	Carbohydrates **60g**	Protein **9g**

the INGREDIENTS

⅓ cup rolled oats

¼ cup quinoa

1¼ cups almond milk

pinch of ground cinnamon

½ banana, sliced

6 blueberries

1 tsp dried cranberries

1 tsp honey

1 tsp pumpkin seeds

the PREP

1 Put the oats and quinoa in a saucepan, then stir in the almond milk and cinnamon. Bring to a boil, then reduce the heat and simmer gently, stirring occasionally, for 15–20 minutes, or until the quinoa is tender. (If it thickens too much, add a little water until it becomes creamy.)

2 Spoon the porridge into a serving bowl, then add the banana, blueberries, and cranberries; drizzle with the honey; and sprinkle the pumpkin seeds over it.

the BUILD

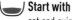 **Start with**
oat and quinoa
porridge

 Add in
banana, blueberries,
and cranberries

 Finish with
honey and
pumpkin seeds

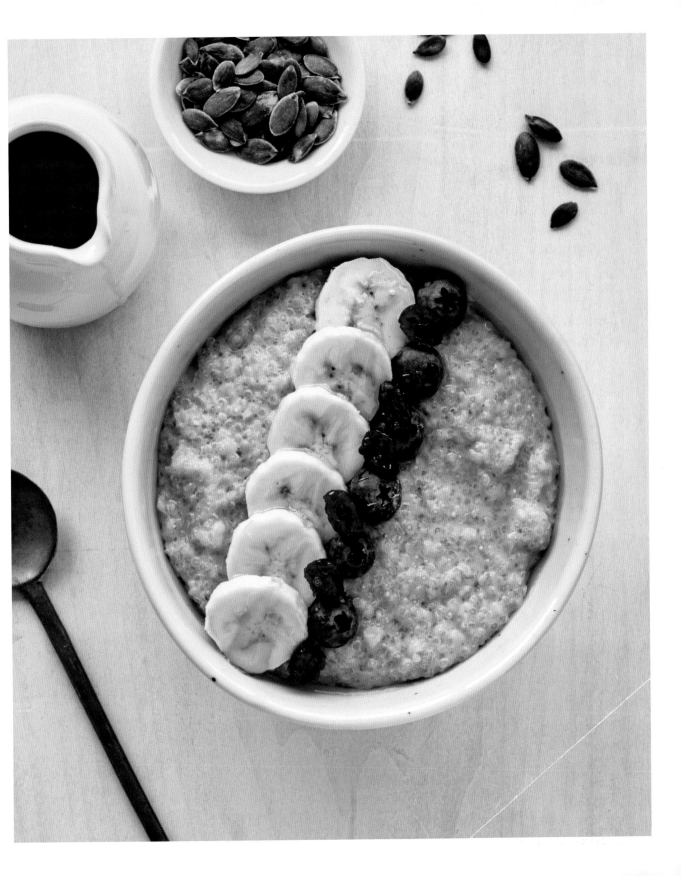

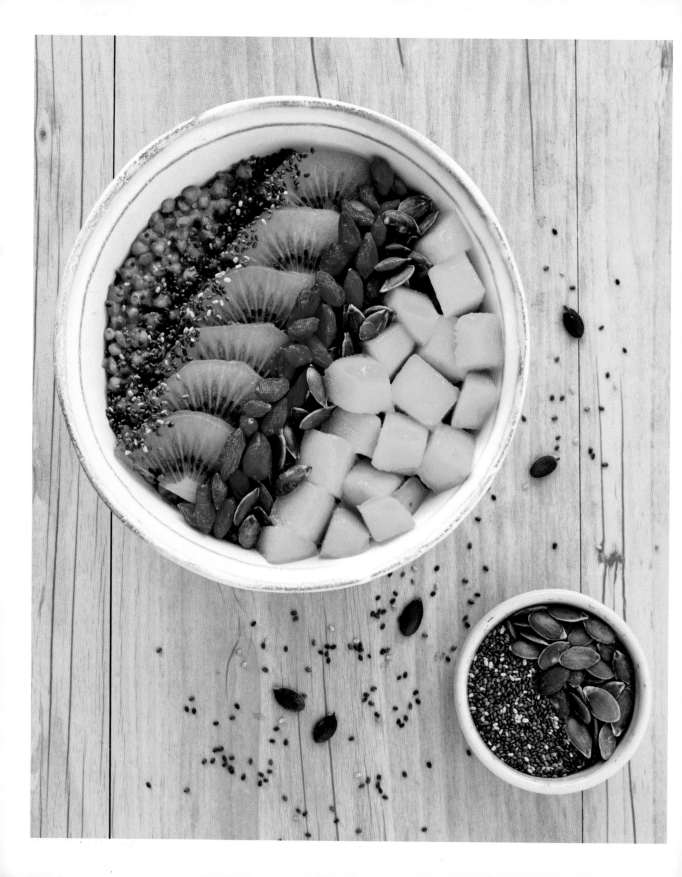

Buckwheat & honey porridge
with tropical fruit & goji

prep **15 MIN**   cook **20 MIN**

Buckwheat is a great replacement for oats in a morning porridge and helps maintain steady blood sugar levels.

Calories **390**	Cholesterol **0mg**	Dietary fiber **6g**
Total fat **9.5g**	Sodium **83mg**	Sugars **26g**
Saturated fat **3.5g**	Carbohydrates **65g**	Protein **8g**

the INGREDIENTS

1 tsp coconut oil

3 tbsp buckwheat

⅔ cup almond milk

pinch of acai powder

pinch of sea salt

1 tsp honey

1 kiwi, peeled and sliced

½ cup mango, cut into cubes

2 tsp dried goji berries

1 tsp pumpkin seeds

1 tsp chia seeds

the PREP

1 Heat the coconut oil in a deep-sided frying pan until it has melted, then stir in the buckwheat, almond milk, and 1⅔ cups of water. Bring to a boil, then reduce the heat to a gentle simmer and stir in the acai powder, sea salt, and honey. Simmer for 15–20 minutes or until the buckwheat is tender. (Add a little hot water if it thickens too much.)

2 Spoon the porridge into a serving bowl, then top with the kiwi, mango, and goji berries, and scatter the pumpkin and chia seeds over it.

the BUILD

 Start with buckwheat and honey porridge

 Add in kiwi, mango, and goji berries

 Finish with pumpkin seeds and chia seeds

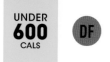

Oat & almond granola
with yogurt & blueberries

prep **5 MIN**   cook **15 MIN**

Making your own granola means you know exactly what's in it, so you can avoid hidden calories and sugars.	Calories **459**	Cholesterol **0mg**	Dietary fiber **5g**

Calories **459**	Cholesterol **0mg**	Dietary fiber **5g**
Total fat **23g**	Sodium **12mg**	Sugars **12g**
Saturated fat **5g**	Carbohydrates **47g**	Protein **13g**

the INGREDIENTS

1 cup rolled oats

2 tsp pumpkin seeds

8 almonds, roughly chopped

1 tsp dried cranberries

1 tsp honey

1 tsp extra virgin olive oil

1 tbsp coconut milk yogurt

10 blueberries

the PREP

1 Preheat the oven to 300°F (150°C). Put the oats, pumpkin seeds, almonds, and dried cranberries in a nonstick roasting pan. Mix the honey and extra virgin olive oil in a small bowl, then pour over the oat mixture and thoroughly combine.

2 Roast for 15 minutes, or until the granola turns golden brown, stirring halfway through. (This makes 2 portions. Once cool, store the extra portion in an airtight container for up to 1 week.)

3 Allow the granola to cool before putting it in a serving bowl, then spoon the coconut milk yogurt over it and serve with the blueberries.

the BUILD

 Start with
oat and almond granola

 Add in
coconut yogurt

 Finish with
blueberries

DF GF

UNDER
600
CALS

Spinach & matcha smoothie
with cashews

prep **5 MIN**   cook **NONE**

This green super-powered drink for the morning is full of iron-rich foods to give you plenty of energy for the day.

Calories **429**	Cholesterol **0mg**	Dietary fiber **4.5g**
Total fat **27g**	Sodium **183mg**	Sugars **15g**
Saturated fat **5g**	Carbohydrates **24g**	Protein **20g**

the INGREDIENTS

½ tsp matcha green tea powder

12 cashews

½ cup silken tofu

1 cup almond milk

2 handfuls of spinach leaves

1½ tsp honey

1 tsp chia seeds

the PREP

1 Mix the matcha powder in a cup with ½ tbsp slightly cooled boiling water. Make the smoothie by blending the cashews in a blender until ground. Add the silken tofu, almond milk, matcha mixture, spinach leaves, and 1 tsp of the honey to the blender and blend on full power until smooth.

2 Pour the smoothie into a serving bowl and let it firm up for 4–5 minutes. (If the smoothie isn't firm enough, put it in the freezer for 15 minutes.) Drizzle with the remaining ½ tsp of honey and sprinkle with the chia seeds.

the BUILD

 Start with
spinach and matcha smoothie

 Add in
honey

 Finish with
chia seeds

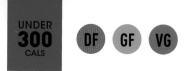

UNDER 300 CALS · **DF** · **GF** · **VG**

Blackberry smoothie
with kiwi & papaya

prep **10 MIN**   cook **NONE**

Blackberries are a low-calorie fruit packed with vitamin C, and they give a vibrant color to this smoothie.

Calories **237**	Cholesterol **0mg**	Dietary fiber **9g**
Total fat **8g**	Sodium **131mg**	Sugars **30g**
Saturated fat **0.8g**	Carbohydrates **32g**	Protein **6g**

the INGREDIENTS

1 cup almond milk

½ cup blackberries, plus 3 extra to serve

½ banana

1 tsp flaxseeds

1 kiwi, sliced

2 papaya slices

1 tsp sunflower seeds

the PREP

1 Make the smoothie by blending the almond milk, blackberries, and banana in a blender until smooth, then add the flaxseeds and blend again until well combined.

2 Pour the smoothie into a serving bowl. (If the smoothie isn't firm enough, put it in the freezer for 15 minutes.) Add the kiwi, papaya, and extra blackberries, and sprinkle the sunflower seeds over it.

the BUILD

 Start with
blackberry and banana smoothie

 Add in
kiwi, papaya, and blackberries

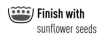 **Finish with**
sunflower seeds

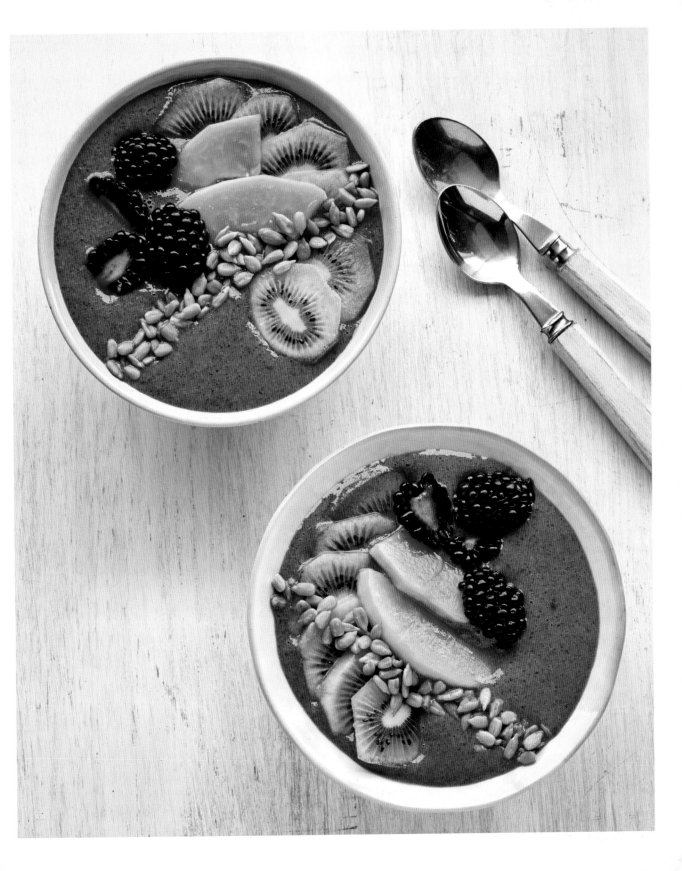

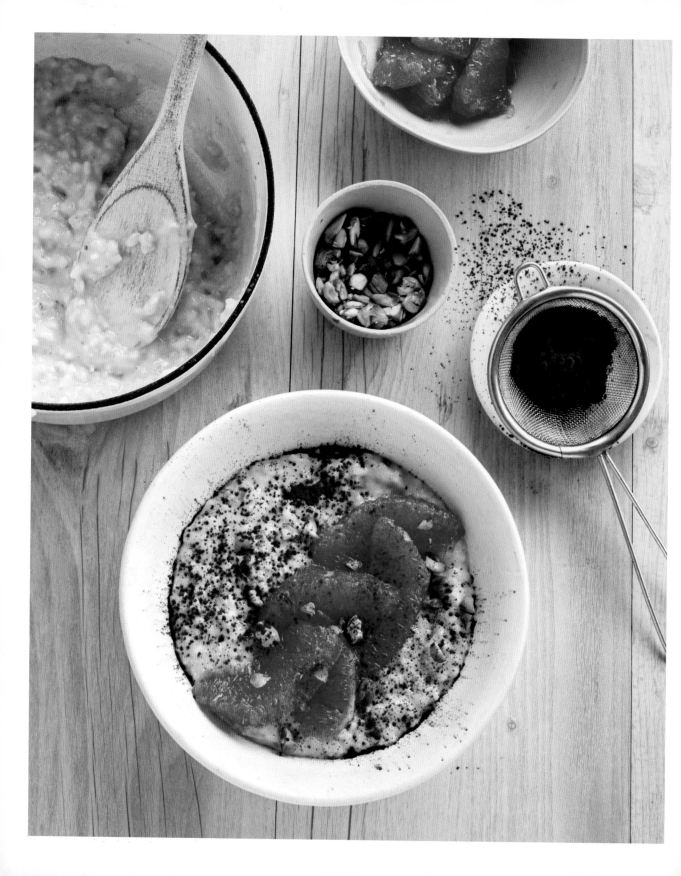

Oat & almond milk porridge
with grapefruit & cocoa

prep **5 MIN** cook **15 MIN**

The beautiful colors of the pink grapefruit and pistachio make this a feast for the eyes and the stomach.

Calories **388**	Cholesterol **0mg**	Dietary fiber **8g**
Total fat **10g**	Sodium **131mg**	Sugars **19g**
Saturated fat **1.5g**	Carbohydrates **59g**	Protein **11g**

the INGREDIENTS

½ cup rolled oats

1 cup almond milk

1 pink grapefruit, peeled and segmented

¼ tsp 70% cocoa powder

1 tsp pistachios, chopped

the PREP

1 Put the oats in a saucepan, then stir in the almond milk and 1 cup of water. Bring to a boil, then reduce the heat to a gentle simmer. Cook for 10–15 minutes, stirring occasionally, or until creamy.

2 Spoon the porridge into a serving bowl, add the grapefruit, and sprinkle the cocoa powder and pistachios over it.

the BUILD

 Start with oat and almond milk porridge

 Add in grapefruit segments

 Finish with cocoa powder and pistachios

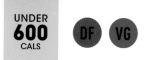

UNDER 600 CALS · DF · VG

Oat & coconut milk muesli
with raspberries

prep **5 MIN**   cook **NONE**

Soaking oats in coconut milk overnight makes for an easily portable breakfast the next morning.

Calories **481**	Cholesterol **0mg**	Dietary fiber **10g**
Total fat **18g**	Sodium **5mg**	Sugars **18g**
Saturated fat **4g**	Carbohydrates **62g**	Protein **13g**

the INGREDIENTS

1 cup rolled oats

1 cup coconut milk drink

1 tsp chia seeds

6 almonds, roughly chopped

1 Gala apple, cored and finely chopped

7 raspberries

the PREP

1 Make the muesli the night before serving, or at least 2 hours before. Put the oats in a bowl, then stir in the coconut milk drink, chia seeds, and almonds, ensuring the oats are completely coated. Cover and refrigerate for 2 hours, or overnight if possible.

2 Spoon the muesli into a serving bowl, then stir in the apple and scatter the raspberries over it.

the BUILD

 Start with oat and coconut milk muesli

 Add in apple

 Finish with raspberries

DF GF

UNDER
600
CALS

Cocoa & quinoa porridge
with strawberries

prep **5 MIN**   cook **20 MIN**

Yes, even a weight loss bowl can have
a little chocolate in it! The quinoa's
protein keeps this meal healthy.

Calories **469**	Cholesterol **0mg**	Dietary fibre **8g**
Total fat **14g**	Sodium **301mg**	Sugars **27g**
Saturated fat **1.5g**	Carbohydrates **64g**	Protein **16g**

the INGREDIENTS

½ cup quinoa

2 cups almond milk

½ tsp cocoa powder

1 tsp honey

3 large strawberries, hulled and sliced

1 tsp almond flakes

1 tsp milled flaxseeds

the PREP

1 Put the quinoa in a saucepan, add the almond milk, and
stir in the cocoa powder and honey. Bring to a boil, then
reduce the heat to a gentle simmer, stirring occasionally,
and cook for 15–20 minutes or until the mixture is
smooth and the quinoa is tender. Let it cool for 1 minute.

2 Spoon the porridge into a serving bowl, then add the
strawberries, almonds, and flaxseeds.

the BUILD

 Start with
quinoa, almond milk,
and cocoa porridge

 Add in
strawberries
and almonds

 Finish with
flaxseeds

Quick-start breakfasts   **41**

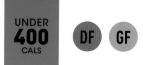

UNDER **400** CALS   DF   GF

Quinoa & honey porridge
with strawberries & papaya

prep **5 MIN**   cook **20 MIN**

Using quinoa to make porridge offers a great alternative to oats, and adding fruit gives each mouthful a sweet pop.

Calories **388**	Cholesterol **0mg**	Dietary fiber **8g**
Total fat **8g**	Sodium **216mg**	Sugars **25g**
Saturated fat **0.7g**	Carbohydrates **62g**	Protein **13g**

the INGREDIENTS

½ cup quinoa

1¼ cups almond milk

1 tsp honey

¼ cup papaya, cubed

¼ cup strawberries, hulled and sliced

1 tsp pomegranate seeds

the PREP

1 Put the quinoa in a saucepan, then pour in the almond milk and honey. Bring to a boil, then reduce the heat to a gentle simmer. Cook for 15–20 minutes, stirring occasionally, or until the quinoa is tender. (If the porridge starts to thicken too much, add a little hot water.)

2 Spoon the porridge into a serving bowl, then add the papaya and strawberries and sprinkle with the pomegranate seeds.

the BUILD

 Start with
quinoa and
honey porridge

 Add in
strawberries
and papaya

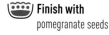 **Finish with**
pomegranate seeds

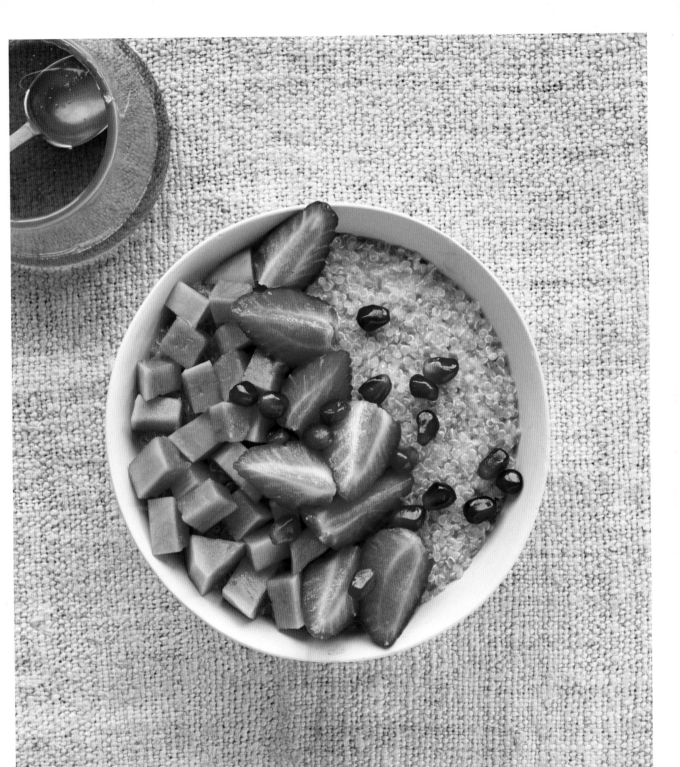

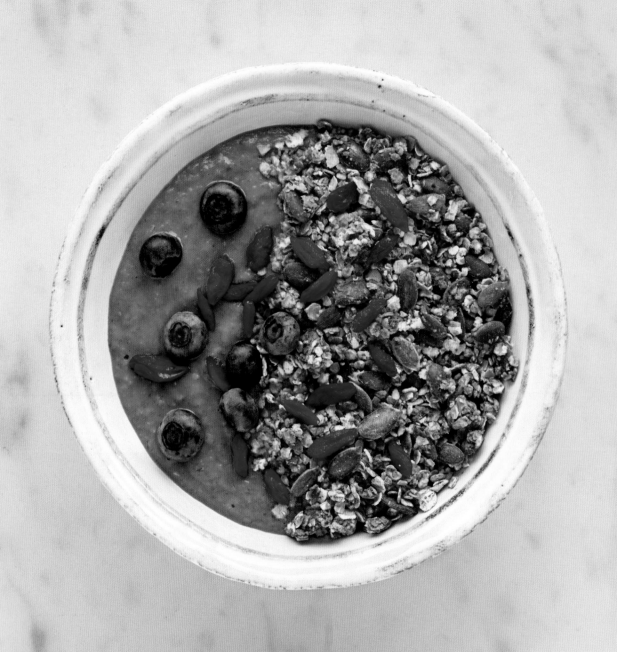

DF UNDER **600** CALS

Kale & orange smoothie
with granola

prep **10 MIN**   cook **15 MIN**

Filled to the brim with nutrient-rich
ingredients, this breakfast smoothie
will really boost your day.

Calories **549**	Cholesterol **0mg**	Dietary fiber **12g**
Total fat **30g**	Sodium **204mg**	Sugars **33g**
Saturated fat **5g**	Carbohydrates **50g**	Protein **14g**

the INGREDIENTS

½ cup rolled oats

¼ cup pumpkin seeds

pinch of ground cinnamon

1½ tsp honey

2 cups kale, coarse stalks removed,
   leaves roughly chopped

1 cup spinach leaves

1 orange, peeled and segmented

1in (2.5cm) piece of fresh ginger, peeled
   and roughly chopped

½ avocado

1⅓ cup almond milk

1 tsp acai powder

2 tsp flaxseeds

8 blueberries

1 tsp goji berries

the PREP

1 Preheat the oven to 400°F (200°C). Combine the oats,
   pumpkin seeds, cinnamon, and 1 tsp of the honey in
   a roasting pan. Roast for 10–15 minutes or until the
   granola is golden brown and crunchy, then set aside until
   cool. (This makes 2 portions. Once cool, store the extra
   portion in an airtight container for up to 3 days.)

2 Make the smoothie by blending the kale, spinach, orange,
   ginger, and avocado in a blender. Add the almond milk and
   blend until well combined. Add the acai powder, flaxseeds,
   and remaining ½ tsp of honey, then blend again until
   smooth. If it's too thick, add a little water and blend again.
   (If the smoothie isn't firm enough, put it in the freezer for
   15 minutes.)

3 Pour the smoothie into a serving bowl, then add the
   granola and sprinkle with the blueberries and goji berries.

the BUILD

 Start with
kale and orange
smoothie

 Add in
oat and pumpkin
seed granola

 Finish with
blueberries
and goji berries

UNDER 600 CALS

DF

Oat & cinnamon porridge
with pear & almonds

prep **5 MIN**   cook **10 MIN**

Almonds complement the pear, while cinnamon adds warmth. Also try apple, toasted hazelnuts, and nutmeg.

Calories **553**	Cholesterol **0mg**	Dietary fiber **9g**
Total fat **22g**	Sodium **255mg**	Sugars **29g**
Saturated fat **2g**	Carbohydrates **70g**	Protein **15g**

the INGREDIENTS

½ cup rolled oats

2 cups almond milk

pinch of ground cinnamon, plus extra to serve

1 tsp honey

½ pear, peeled, cored, and sliced lengthwise

8 whole almonds

the PREP

1 Put the oats in a saucepan, pour in the almond milk, then add the cinnamon and honey. Bring to a boil, then reduce the heat to a gentle simmer. Cook for 5–7 minutes, stirring occasionally, or until thick and creamy. Allow to cool for 1–2 minutes.

2 Spoon the porridge into a serving bowl. Add the pear and almonds and sprinkle a little cinnamon over it.

the BUILD

 Start with
oat and cinnamon porridge

 Add in
pear and almonds

 Finish with
cinnamon

DF

UNDER
400
CALS

Buckwheat & acai porridge
with fig

prep **5 MIN**   cook **20 MIN**

This porridge contains two great superfoods—buckwheat and acai—both enhanced by sweeter ingredients.

Calories **400**	Cholesterol **0mg**	Dietary fiber **2g**
Total fat **9g**	Sodium **253mg**	Sugars **21g**
Saturated fat **1g**	Carbohydrates **70g**	Protein **9g**

the INGREDIENTS

½ cup buckwheat

2 cups almond milk

1 tsp honey

1 tsp acai powder

1 tsp pumpkin seeds

1 small fig, halved

the PREP

1 Put the buckwheat in a saucepan, then stir in the almond milk, honey, and acai powder. Bring to a boil, then reduce the heat to a gentle simmer and cook for 15–20 minutes, stirring occasionally, or until the buckwheat is tender. Stir in the acai powder, remove the saucepan from the heat, and allow to cool for 1 minute.

2 Spoon the porridge into a serving bowl. Sprinkle over the pumpkin seeds and top with the fig halves.

the BUILD

 Start with
buckwheat
and acai porridge

 Add in
pumpkin seeds

 Finish with
fig

UNDER
600
CALS

Matcha & banana smoothie
with almonds

prep **15 MIN**   cook **NONE**

This is a bowl full of healthy goodness:
a smoothie topped with fruit, nuts,
and seeds... and no cooking needed.

Calories **450**	Cholesterol **0.1mg**	Dietary fiber **5g**
Total fat **21g**	Sodium **89mg**	Sugars **27g**
Saturated fat **2g**	Carbohydrates **49g**	Protein **14g**

the INGREDIENTS

1 tsp matcha green tea powder

½ cup almond milk

2 tbsp rolled oats

½ banana

1 tsp honey

2 tsp 0% fat plain Greek yogurt

2 strawberries, hulled and sliced

1 passion fruit, halved and seeds
  removed

1 tsp flaxseeds

⅓ cup blanched almonds, chopped

the PREP

1 Mix the matcha powder in a cup with 1 tbsp slightly cooled
boiling water. Blend the almond milk and oats in a blender.
Add the matcha mix, banana, honey, and Greek yogurt and
blend again until well combined. (If the smoothie isn't firm
enough, put it in the freezer for 15 minutes.)

2 Pour the smoothie into a serving bowl, then add the
strawberries, passion fruit seeds, flaxseeds, and almonds.

the BUILD

 Start with
matcha and
banana smoothie

 Add in
strawberries
and passion fruit

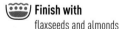 **Finish with**
flaxseeds and almonds

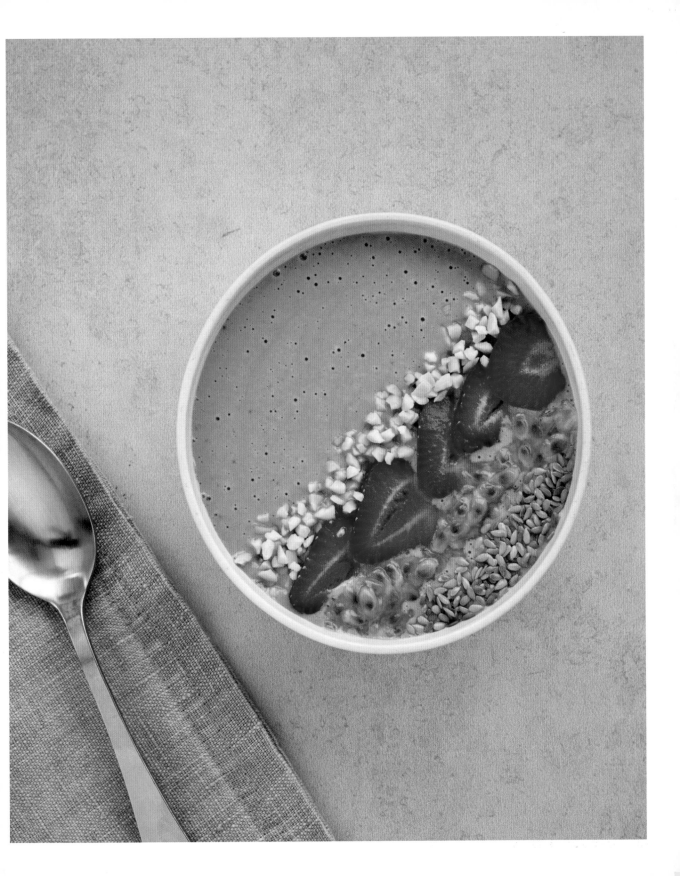

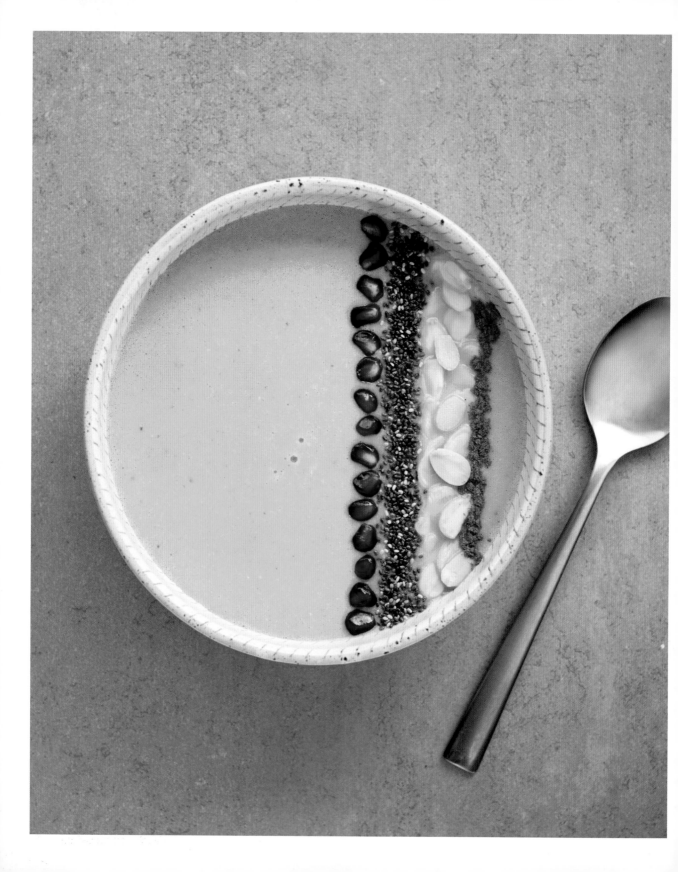

DF **VG** **UNDER 400 CALS**

Oat, orange & carrot smoothie
with almonds

prep **10 MIN**   cook **NONE**

Bright colors and flavors make this bowl appealing, while the nutrients will have you bouncing all morning.

Calories **323**	Cholesterol **0mg**	Dietary fiber **10g**
Total fat **9g**	Sodium **158mg**	Sugars **36g**
Saturated fat **1g**	Carbohydrates **48g**	Protein **7g**

the INGREDIENTS

1 tbsp rolled oats

1 orange, peeled and segmented

1 carrot, roughly chopped

1 cup almond milk

2 dates, roughly chopped

1 tsp almond flakes

1 tsp chia seeds

ground cinnamon

1 tsp pomegranate seeds

the PREP

1 Process the oats, orange, carrot, almond milk, and dates in a blender until smooth. (If the smoothie isn't firm enough, put it in the freezer for 15 minutes.)

2 Pour the smoothie into a serving bowl, then add the almond flakes and chia seeds and sprinkle with ground cinnamon and the pomegranate seeds.

the BUILD

 Start with
oat, orange, and carrot smoothie

 Add in
almond flakes and chia seeds

 Finish with
ground cinnamon and pomegranate seeds

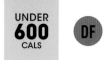

UNDER 600 CALS · **DF**

Oat & acai porridge
with blackberries & hemp

prep **5 MIN**   cook **15 MIN**

This bowl has plenty of antioxidants, especially in the acai and blackberries, and makes a delicious breakfast.

Calories **469**	Cholesterol **0mg**	Dietary fiber **8g**
Total fat **14g**	Sodium **301mg**	Sugars **27g**
Saturated fat **1.5g**	Carbohydrates **64g**	Protein **16g**

the INGREDIENTS

½ cup rolled oats

1 cup almond milk

pinch of sea salt

1 tsp acai powder

pinch of freshly grated nutmeg

8 blackberries

1 tsp ground hemp seeds

½ tsp honey

the PREP

1 Put the oats in a saucepan, then pour in the almond milk. Add the salt, acai powder, and nutmeg. Bring to a boil, then reduce the heat to a gentle simmer. Cook for 10–15 minutes, stirring occasionally, until the porridge is thick and creamy. Allow to cool for 1 minute.

2 Spoon the porridge into a serving bowl. Top with the blackberries and hemp seeds, and finish with a drizzle of honey.

the BUILD

 Start with
oat and acai porridge

 Add in
blackberries and hemp seeds

 Finish with
honey

DF VG

UNDER
400
CALS

Date & cocoa smoothie
with chia seeds

prep **5 MIN**   cook **NONE**

Cocoa powder adds a bitter edge to this sweet smoothie, while the apricots provide plenty of fiber.

Calories **350**	Cholesterol **0mg**	Dietary fiber **8g**
Total fat **6.5g**	Sodium **140mg**	Sugars **46g**
Saturated fat **1g**	Carbohydrates **62g**	Protein **7g**

the INGREDIENTS

5 dates, pitted

¾ cup rolled oats

½ tsp dark cocoa powder

1 cup almond milk

3 dried apricots, roughly chopped

1 tsp chia seeds

the PREP

1 Make the smoothie by putting the dates, oats, cocoa powder, and almond milk into a blender and blending until well combined. (If the smoothie isn't firm enough, put it in the freezer for 15 minutes.)

2 Pour the smoothie into a serving bowl, then add the apricots and finish with the chia seeds.

the BUILD

 Start with
date and cocoa smoothie

 Add in
apricots

 Finish with
chia seeds

Weekend brunch

These bowls offer healthier, more streamlined takes on classic mid-morning meals and are bursting with bold flavors and savory indulgence, but easy on the waistline.

Rice & smoked haddock
with pineapple salsa

prep **15 MIN**   cook **20 MIN**

The sweetness of the salsa contrasts wonderfully with the subtle smokiness of the haddock and vibrant spinach.

Calories **482**	Cholesterol **74mg**	Dietary fiber **6g**
Total fat **6g**	Sodium **679mg**	Sugars **10g**
Saturated fat **3.5g**	Carbohydrates **70g**	Protein **35g**

the INGREDIENTS

⅓ cup basmati rice

¼ cup reduced-fat coconut milk

sea salt and freshly ground black pepper

2¼oz (70g) undyed smoked haddock

pinch of medium curry powder (optional)

½ cup spinach leaves

1 green onion, green part only, finely sliced

¼ red chili pepper, sliced

For the salsa

⅓ cup fresh pineapple, cut into cubes

pinch of nigella seeds

handful of cilantro leaves, finely chopped

the PREP

1 Put the basmati rice into a saucepan, pour in the coconut milk and ¼ cup of water, and season with a pinch of sea salt. Cook with the lid on for 10–12 minutes or until the liquid has been absorbed and the rice is tender. Set aside, leaving the lid on.

2 Put the haddock in a deep-sided frying pan and cover with cold water, then add the curry powder (if using). Bring to a boil, then reduce the heat to a gentle simmer, cover and cook for 5–6 minutes or until the fish is cooked. Carefully remove the fish using a spatula and set aside.

3 Meanwhile, steam the spinach over boiling water until the leaves wilt.

4 Make the salsa by mixing the pineapple, nigella seeds, and cilantro leaves in a bowl, then season with salt and pepper. Set aside.

5 Fluff up the rice using a fork, and spoon it into a serving bowl, then add the haddock and spinach, spoon on the salsa, and sprinkle the green onion and red chili pepper.

the BUILD

 Start with
rice, haddock, and spinach leaves

 Add in
pineapple salsa

 Finish with
green onion and red chili pepper

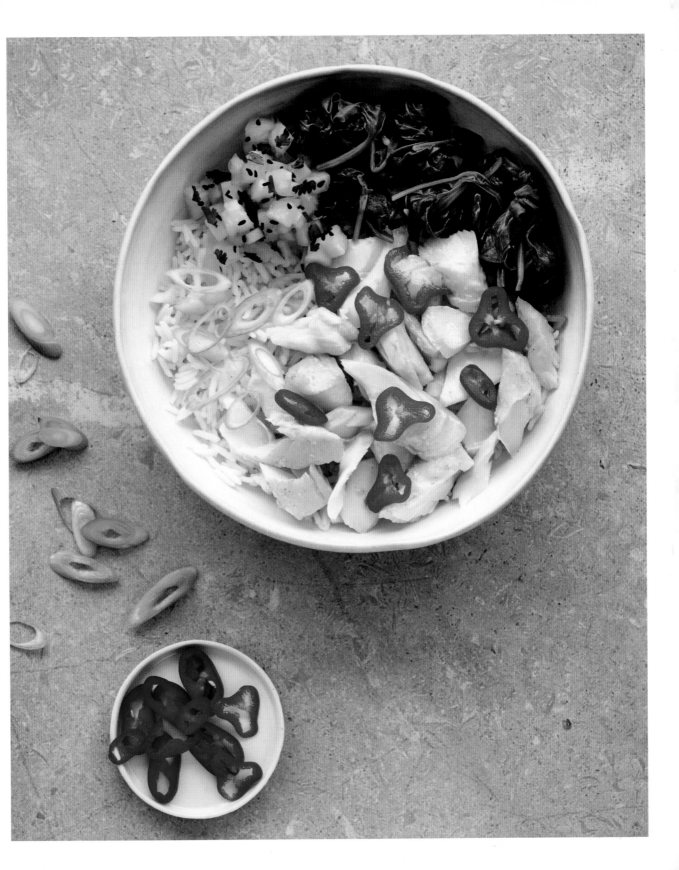

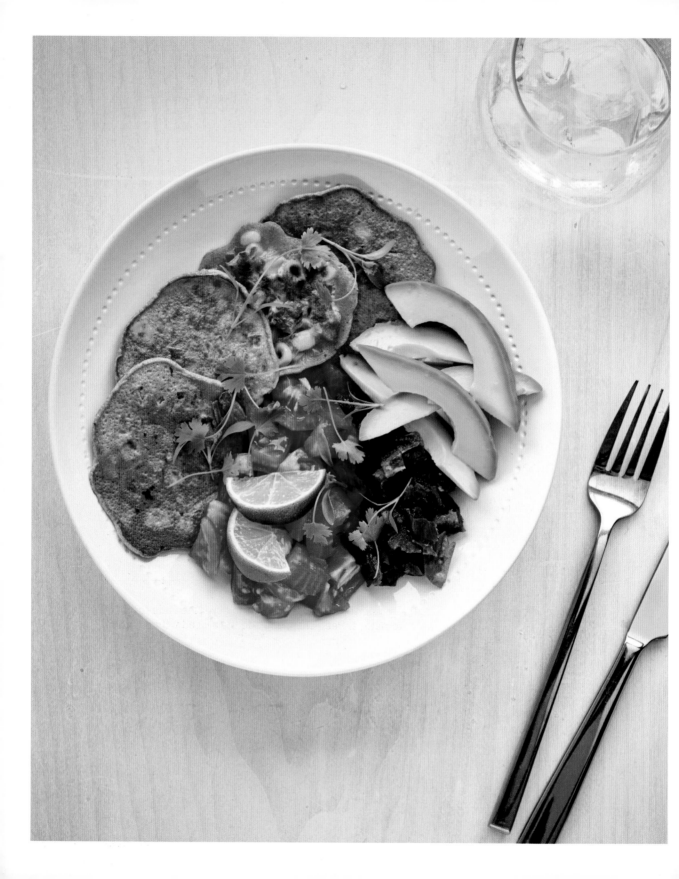

Corn & red pepper fritters
with avocado & dates

prep **15 MIN**   cook **10 MIN**

These buckwheat fritters take only minutes to cook, and they pair well with creamy avocado and sweet dates.

Calories **487**	Cholesterol **214mg**	Dietary fiber **8g**
Total fat **32g**	Sodium **113g**	Sugars **17g**
Saturated fat **6g**	Carbohydrates **32g**	Protein **13g**

the INGREDIENTS

2 tbsp sweet corn

⅓ cup red bell pepper, finely chopped

2 tbsp buckwheat flour, or other gluten-free flour

pinch of red pepper flakes

a few cilantro leaves, finely chopped

1 egg, lightly beaten

1 tbsp almond milk

sea salt and freshly ground black pepper

2 tomatoes

1 tbsp olive oil

½ avocado

2 dates, pitted and sliced

handful of flat-leaf parsley (optional)

lime wedges (optional)

the PREP

1 Make the fritters by mixing the sweet corn, red bell pepper, buckwheat flour, red pepper flakes, cilantro leaves, egg, and almond milk in a bowl. Season with salt and pepper and set aside.

2 Cut a cross on the base of each tomato and put into a bowl of boiling water for 20 seconds. Transfer to a bowl of cold water, peel off and discard their skins, roughly chop them, and set aside.

3 Heat the olive oil in a nonstick frying pan over medium heat, swirling it to coat the pan. Add 1 tablespoon of the batter to the pan, then repeat to make 4 fritters, leaving a little space between each. Leave them undisturbed for 3 minutes or until the underside starts to turn golden brown. Use a spatula to carefully turn them, cooking the other side for the same time, or until golden brown.

4 Transfer the fritters to a serving bowl, then add the tomatoes. Peel, chop, and add the avocado, then the dates. Sprinkle with the parsley and finish with lime wedges to squeeze over (if using).

the BUILD

 Start with
sweet corn and red pepper fritters

 Add in
tomatoes, avocado, and dates

 Finish with
flat-leaf parsley and lime wedges

UNDER 600 CALS · DF · GF

Sweet potato fritters
with bean sprouts

prep **15 MIN**   cook **25 MIN**

This substantial brunch gives you slow-burning energy—exactly what you need from a bowl in the morning.

Calories **430**	Cholesterol **213mg**	Dietary fiber **11g**
Total fat **12g**	Sodium **253mg**	Sugars **16g**
Saturated fat **2.5g**	Carbohydrates **59g**	Protein **16g**

the INGREDIENTS

1 sweet potato, peeled and grated

2 green onions, finely chopped

finely grated zest of ½ lemon

pinch of red pepper flakes

sea salt and freshly ground black pepper

1 egg, lightly beaten

1 tbsp rice flour, or other gluten-free flour

1 tsp milled flaxseeds

½ tsp olive oil

¼ red onion, sliced

1 tsp rice vinegar

1 tsp chopped chives

1 cup bean sprouts

handful of watercress

a few basil leaves (optional)

For the dressing

1 tsp extra virgin olive oil

½ tsp white wine vinegar

½ tsp Dijon mustard

the PREP

1 Preheat the oven to 400°F (200°C) and combine the sweet potato, green onions, lemon zest, and red pepper flakes in a bowl, seasoning with salt and pepper. Mix in the egg, rice flour, and flaxseeds. Form half the mixture into a ball, then flatten it into a fritter shape. Make another fritter with the remaining mixture.

2 Brush a baking sheet with the olive oil, then place the fritters on the sheet. Bake for 10–15 minutes, then flip them and bake on the other side for another 10 minutes, or until they start to turn golden brown on both sides.

3 Meanwhile, make the dressing by mixing the extra virgin olive oil, white wine vinegar, and Dijon mustard in a bowl, seasoning with salt and pepper. Set aside.

4 Mix the red onion, rice vinegar, and chives in a bowl.

5 Places the fritters in a serving bowl, then add the red onion mixture, bean sprouts, and watercress. Drizzle with the dressing and scatter with the basil leaves (if using).

the BUILD

 Start with sweet potato fritters

 Add in red onion, bean sprouts, and watercress

 Finish with Dijon mustard dressing and basil leaves

DF **GF**

UNDER 600 CALS

Roasted sardines & tomatoes
with avocado & apple

prep **5 MIN**   cook **20 MIN**

Sardines are an excellent source of B$_{12}$ and omega-3 fatty acids, and taste great with tomatoes and spinach.

Calories **410**	Cholesterol **244mg**	Dietary fiber **6g**
Total fat **30g**	Sodium **199mg**	Sugars **8g**
Saturated fat **7g**	Carbohydrates **9g**	Protein **24g**

the INGREDIENTS

1 tsp olive oil

3 sardine fillets, about 1½ oz (40g) each

sea salt and freshly ground black pepper

6 cherry tomatoes

1 egg

2 cups spinach leaves

½ avocado

½ Gala apple, cored, and finely sliced

juice of ½ lemon

pinch of sesame seeds

pinch of chopped chives

the PREP

1 Preheat the oven to 400°F (200°C). Lightly coat a roasting pan with ½ tsp of the olive oil. Add the sardines to the pan, and season with salt and pepper. Toss the cherry tomatoes with the remaining ½ tsp of olive oil, then add them to the pan. Season again, then roast for 10–15 minutes, or until the sardines are cooked through and begin to turn golden brown. Set aside.

2 Meanwhile, put the egg into a saucepan with enough cold water to cover, bring to a boil, and cook for 5 minutes, then drain, and cover with cold water. Once the egg is cool enough to handle, peel and halve it.

3 Steam the spinach for 1 minute or until wilted.

4 Chop the avocado, put it in a bowl and season with salt and pepper, then mix in the apple and lemon juice.

5 Transfer the spinach and sardines to a serving bowl, then add the egg. Spoon in the tomatoes and the avocado mixture, and sprinkle with the sesame seeds and chives.

the BUILD

 Start with
tomatoes
and sardines

 Add in
egg, spinach,
avocado, and apple

 Finish with
sesame seeds
and chives

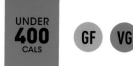
Sweet potato & cabbage hash
with dukkah

prep **15 MIN**   cook **30 MIN**

A pinch of dukkah and a zing of lemon zest brighten the flavors in this healthy version of a breakfast hash.

Calories **310**	Cholesterol **0mg**	Dietary fiber **14g**
Total fat **4g**	Sodium **105mg**	Sugars **21.5g**
Saturated fat **0.7g**	Carbohydrates **55g**	Protein **6g**

the INGREDIENTS

1½ cups sweet potato, peeled and cubed

sea salt and freshly ground black pepper

1¼ cups cabbage, shredded

1 tsp olive oil

1in (2.5cm) piece of fresh ginger, peeled and finely chopped

1 garlic clove, finely chopped

2 tsp dukkah

finely grated zest of ½ lemon

¼ red onion, finely diced

¼ red chili pepper, finely sliced

1 green onion, green part only, finely sliced

lemon wedges (optional)

the PREP

1   Place the sweet potato in a saucepan of salted cold water to cover. Bring to a boil, cook for 10–15 minutes or until tender, then drain. Set aside.

2   Meanwhile, steam the cabbage over boiling water for 5 minutes, or until softened but still retaining a bite.

3   Heat the olive oil in a nonstick frying pan over medium heat, then add the ginger and garlic. Cook for a few seconds, being careful not to burn them, then stir in the dukkah. Add the sweet potato and cabbage, stirring well, and season with salt and pepper. Continue cooking for 6–8 minutes, or until the hash starts to turn golden brown, stirring occasionally. Add the lemon zest and red onion, combining well.

4   Transfer the sweet potato and cabbage hash to a serving bowl, then sprinkle with the red chili pepper and green onion, and add the lemon wedges (if using), to squeeze over the hash.

the BUILD

 Start with
sweet potato
and cabbage hash

 Add in
red chili pepper
and green onion

 Finish with
lemon wedges

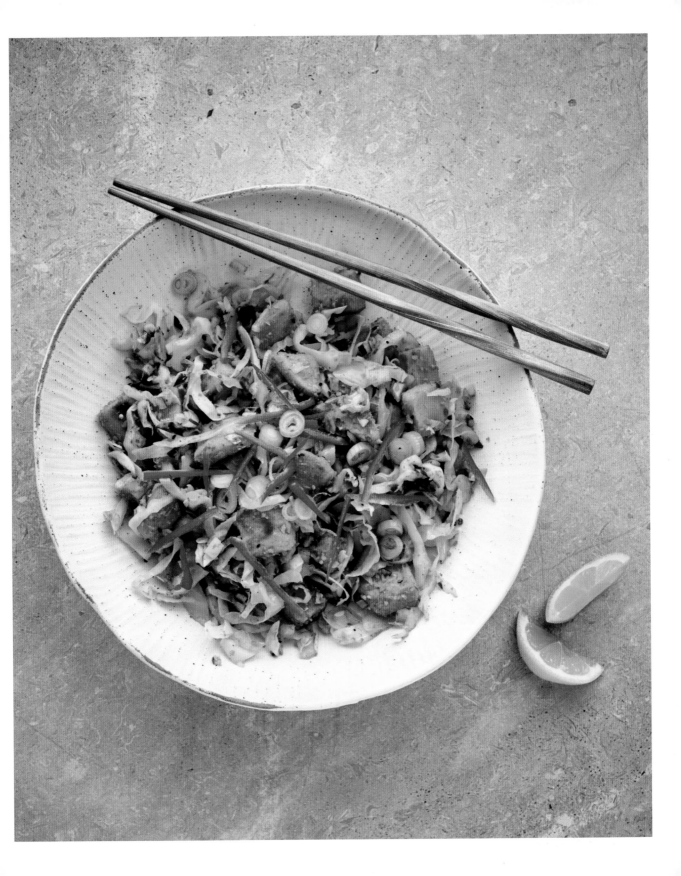

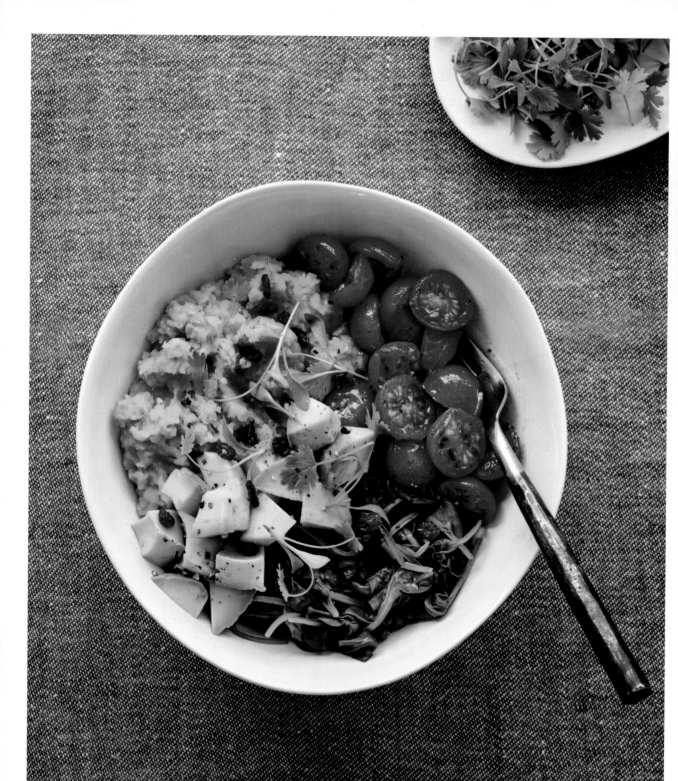

UNDER 600 CALS

Red lentils & cherry tomatoes
with spinach

prep **5 MIN**   cook **15 MIN**

This bowl makes a substantial brunch: hearty red lentils with a pinch of red pepper flakes to liven them up.

Calories **479**	Cholesterol **0mg**	Dietary fiber **12g**
Total fat **20g**	Sodium **124mg**	Sugars **8g**
Saturated fat **4g**	Carbohydrates **48g**	Protein **22g**

the INGREDIENTS

1 tsp dried barberries

⅓ cup red lentils, washed

sea salt and freshly ground black pepper

pinch of red pepper flakes

⅓ cup cherry tomatoes, halved

pinch of sumac

1 tsp olive oil

2½ oz (70g) spinach leaves
(⅓ cup cooked)

½ avocado

pinch of chopped flat-leaf parsley
(optional)

the PREP

1 Put the barberries in a cup, cover with water, and leave to soak for 10 minutes, then drain.

2 Put the red lentils in a saucepan with ⅔ cup water, and some salt and pepper. Bring to a boil, then reduce the heat and simmer gently for 10 minutes or until the lentils are tender, topping off with hot water if the pan starts to dry out. Remove from the heat, stir in the red pepper flakes, and set aside.

3 Meanwhile, heat a griddle pan over medium heat, then toss the tomatoes with the sumac and olive oil in a bowl, seasoning with salt and pepper. Add the tomatoes to the pan and cook for 3–4 minutes, turning halfway through, or until they're lightly charred on both sides.

4 Quickly wilt the spinach in a saucepan, then drain in a sieve, pushing out the excess liquid with the back of a spoon.

5 Transfer the lentils to a serving bowl, then add the tomato mixture and spinach. Chop the avocado and put on top with the barberries, flat-leaf parsley (if using), and black pepper.

the BUILD

 Start with
red lentils

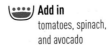 **Add in**
tomatoes, spinach,
and avocado

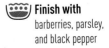 **Finish with**
barberries, parsley,
and black pepper

Quinoa & sweet potatoes
with jeweled yogurt

prep **10 MIN**   cook **20 MIN**

Dried berries and pomegranate seeds
perk up the yogurt, adding sweetness
and crunch to a refreshing brunch.

Calories **453**	Cholesterol **0mg**	Dietary fiber **12g**
Total fat **6.5g**	Sodium **148mg**	Sugars **24.5g**
Saturated fat **1g**	Carbohydrates **78g**	Protein **15g**

the INGREDIENTS

1 tsp barberries

1 tsp goji berries

1 sweet potato, peeled and cubed

1 tsp olive oil

pinch of sumac

sea salt and freshly ground black pepper

2 cups spinach leaves

½ cup quinoa

1 tomato, halved, seeds removed,
  chopped into small pieces

2 tbsp 0% fat plain Greek yogurt

1 tsp pumpkin seeds

1 tsp pomegranate seeds

a few cilantro leaves

the PREP

1 Put the barberries and goji berries into 2 separate cups,
   cover with water, and leave to soak for 10 minutes. Drain.

2 Meanwhile, preheat the oven to 400°F (200°C) and put the
   sweet potato, olive oil, and sumac in a roasting pan, then
   season with salt and pepper. Roast for 15–20 minutes or
   until the sweet potato is tender and golden brown.
   Remove from the oven, stir in the spinach, and
   set aside.

3 At the same time, put the quinoa in a saucepan with
   1 cup of water. Bring to a boil, then reduce the heat to
   a gentle simmer, cover, and cook for 15–20 minutes.
   Remove from the heat.

4 Spoon the quinoa into a serving bowl, then add the
   sweet potato and spinach mixture, tomato, and Greek
   yogurt. Sprinkle over the barberries, goji berries,
   pumpkin seeds, and pomegranate seeds, then finish
   by scattering the cilantro leaves on top.

the BUILD

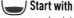 **Start with**
sweet potato
and spinach
mixture, and quinoa

Add in
barberries, goji berries,
pumpkin seeds, and
pomegranate seeds

 Finish with
cilantro leaves

DF GF **UNDER 400 CALS**

Haddock & noodles
with chili salsa

prep **10 MIN**   cook **20 MIN**

This Asian-style bowl provides a great weekend brunch, and the salsa gives you all the spiciness you'll need.

Calories **387**	Cholesterol **54mg**	Dietary fiber **10g**
Total fat **2g**	Sodium **108mg**	Sugars **14g**
Saturated fat **0.7g**	Carbohydrates **57g**	Protein **31g**

the INGREDIENTS

4 oz (110g) haddock, skinned

sea salt and freshly ground black pepper

1 cup vermicelli noodles

1 tsp olive oil

½ red onion, finely sliced

1 tsp tamarind paste

1 large carrot, peeled into ribbons with a vegetable peeler

½ cup peas

a few cilantro leaves

For the salsa

½ red chili pepper, seeds removed, flesh finely chopped

1 tomato, halved, seeds removed, and flesh diced

1 tsp rice vinegar

the PREP

1 Preheat the oven to 375°F (190°C). Place the haddock in a roasting pan, season with salt and pepper, and cover the pan with foil. Bake for 12–15 minutes or until cooked through. Set aside.

2 Meanwhile, add the vermicelli noodles to a bowl, then cover with boiling water. Leave for 5 minutes, or according to the package instructions, then drain.

3 Make the salsa by mixing the red chili pepper, tomato, and rice vinegar in a bowl, seasoning the salsa with salt and pepper.

4 Heat the olive oil in a wok or a frying pan over medium heat, then add the red onion and cook for 3 minutes. Add the tamarind paste and 2 tsp of water, stirring to combine. Add the noodles, tossing to coat completely. Add the carrot and peas and toss again.

5 Transfer the noodles to a serving bowl, then add the fish, spoon in the salsa, and scatter the cilantro leaves.

the BUILD

 Start with
vermicelli noodle mixture

 Add in
roast haddock

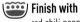 **Finish with**
red chili pepper salsa and cilantro leaves

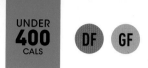

UNDER 400 CALS DF GF

Mackerel & curried rice
with soft-boiled egg

prep **10 MIN**   cook **30 MIN**

This is a deconstructed kedgeree, an Anglo-Indian fish dish that's full of gutsy flavors and ideal for a brunch.

Calories **357**	Cholesterol **220mg**	Dietary fiber **8g**
Total fat **9g**	Sodium **142mg**	Sugars **8g**
Saturated fat **2g**	Carbohydrates **48g**	Protein **17g**

the INGREDIENTS

¼ cup quick-cook brown rice

2 tsp medium curry powder

sea salt and freshly ground black pepper

2 tomatoes, halved, seeds removed, and flesh chopped

1 tsp rice vinegar

2 tbsp peas, defrosted if frozen

handful of flat-leaf parsley, finely chopped

2 oz (60g) smoked mackerel, skinned and roughly shredded

1 egg

¼ green chili pepper, finely sliced (optional)

a few cilantro leaves (optional)

lemon wedge (optional)

the PREP

1 Put the rice, curry powder, and ½ cup of water in a saucepan, then season with salt and pepper. Cover and cook for 20–30 minutes, or until the rice is tender and all the water has been absorbed. Set aside, leaving the lid on.

2 Mix the tomatoes and rice vinegar in a bowl, season with salt and pepper to taste, and set aside.

3 Add half the peas and all the flat-leaf parsley to the rice and combine well.

4 Meanwhile, put the egg into a saucepan with enough cold water to cover, bring to a boil, and cook for 5 minutes, then drain, and place in cold water. Once the egg is cool enough to handle, peel and halve it.

5 Transfer the curried rice to a serving bowl, then add the mackerel, the remaining 1 tbsp of peas, the egg, and the tomatoes. Sprinkle with the green chili pepper and cilantro leaves (if using) and add the lemon wedge (if using), to squeeze over the bowl.

the BUILD

 Start with
curried rice mixture

 Add in
mackerel, peas, egg, and tomatoes

 Finish with
green chili pepper, cilantro leaves, and lemon wedge

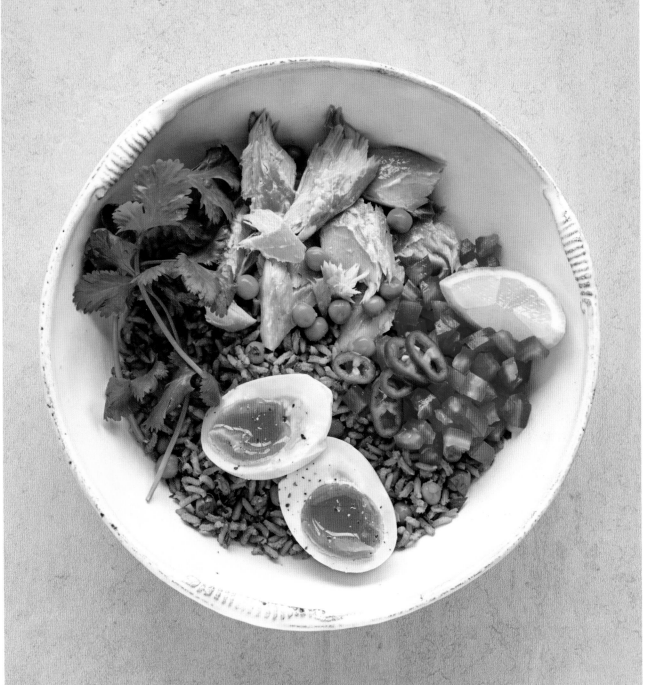

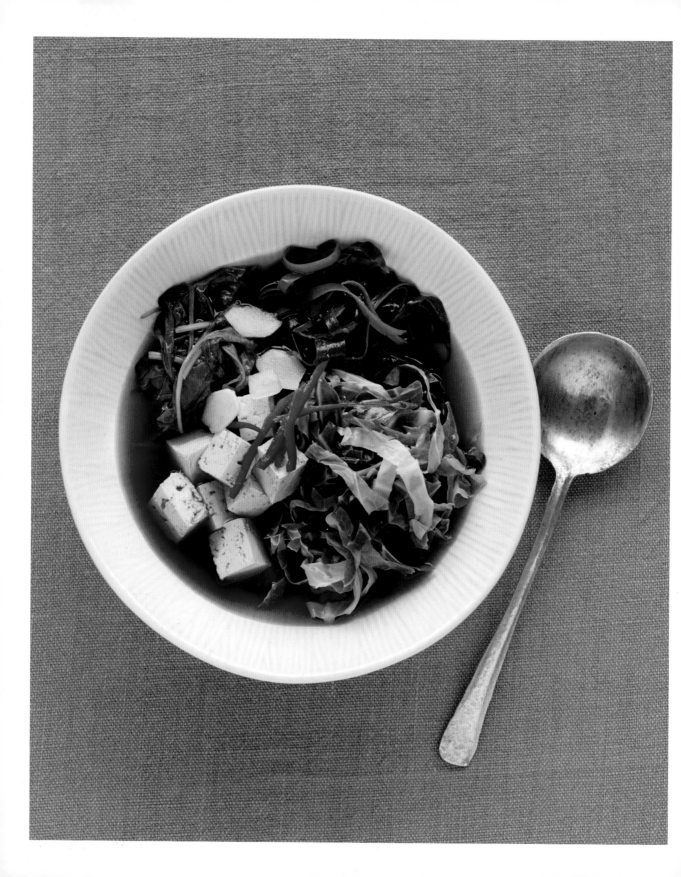

DF **VG** UNDER **300** CALS

Miso broth
with tofu & wakame

prep **10 MIN**   cook **10 MIN**

Wakame is an edible seaweed that's tasty and rich in nutrients, and also very low in calories.

Calories **116**	Cholesterol **0mg**	Dietary fiber **8g**
Total fat **4g**	Sodium **413mg**	Sugars **6g**
Saturated fat **0.5g**	Carbohydrates **7g**	Protein **9g**

the INGREDIENTS

2 pieces of dried wakame seaweed

⅓ cup spinach leaves

½ cup cabbage, shredded

1 tbsp brown rice miso

2 in (5cm) piece of fresh ginger, half grated, half finely sliced

¼ cup firm tofu, chopped into cubes

sea salt and freshly ground black pepper

juice of 1 lemon

½ green onion, finely sliced

¼ red chili pepper, finely sliced

the PREP

1 Place the wakame in a bowl and cover with hot water. Soak for 10 minutes, then drain and shred.

2 Meanwhile, steam the spinach and cabbage over boiling water for 3 minutes.

3 Pour 1 cup of boiling water in a saucepan, then stir in the miso paste with a fork for 2 minutes, or until it starts to dissolve. Bring to a boil, then reduce the heat to a gentle simmer and cook for 1 minute.

4 Add the grated ginger and tofu. Slowly pour in up to ½ cup of boiling water, tasting as you go and stopping when it tastes good to you (be careful not to dilute the miso too much). Season with salt and pepper to taste, then simmer for 5 more minutes.

5 Add the spinach, cabbage, and wakame to a serving bowl, then ladle in the miso broth and tofu. Add a squeeze of lemon juice and sprinkle with the sliced ginger, green onion, and red chili pepper.

the BUILD

 Start with
wakame, spinach, and cabbage

 Add in
miso broth, tofu, and lemon juice

 Finish with
ginger, green onion, and red chili pepper

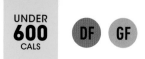

UNDER 600 CALS · DF · GF

Vietnamese shrimp pancake
with chili sauce

prep **10 MIN**   cook **10 MIN**

Known as bánh xèo—"sizzling cake"—this pancake is a Vietnamese staple. Now you can also make it yours.

Calories **570**	Cholesterol **86mg**	Dietary fiber **5.5g**
Total fat **17g**	Sodium **362mg**	Sugars **6g**
Saturated fat **9g**	Carbohydrates **83.5g**	Protein **19g**

the INGREDIENTS

¼ red chili pepper, finely chopped

1 tsp rice vinegar

sea salt and freshly ground black pepper

2 tsp olive oil

1 cup bean sprouts

½ cooked shrimp

½ red bell pepper, finely sliced

handful of cilantro leaves

½ green onion, green part only, finely sliced

2 lime wedges (optional)

For the batter

½ cup rice flour, or other gluten-free flour

1 tsp ground turmeric

¼ cup reduced-fat coconut milk

1 green onion, finely chopped

the PREP

1 Mix the red chili pepper and rice vinegar in a bowl and season with salt and pepper. Set aside.

2 Make the batter by mixing the rice flour and turmeric in a bowl and seasoning with salt and pepper. Add the coconut milk and 1 cup of water and whisk until the batter becomes smooth. Stir in the green onion. (This makes enough batter for 2 pancakes. You can store the extra batter in an airtight container in the fridge for up to 2 days.)

3 Heat 1 tsp of the olive oil in a nonstick frying pan on medium heat. Pour in half the batter, swirling it around the pan to cover the surface. Cook on high, undisturbed, for about 4 minutes on each side, or until it's crispy and the edges begin to come away easily from the sides of the pan.

4 Pile in the bean sprouts, shrimp, and red bell pepper, and fold the pancake over.

5 Use a spatula to transfer the pancake to a serving bowl, then sprinkle with the cilantro leaves and green onion. Spoon on the chili sauce and add the lime wedges (if using) to squeeze over the pancake.

the BUILD

 Start with
stuffed pancake

 Add in
coriander leaves and spring onion

 Finish with
chilli sauce and lime wedges

DF GF VG

UNDER
300
CALS

Kale & scrambled tofu
with mushrooms

prep **5 MIN**   cook **15 MIN**

Who needs eggs when low-calorie silken tofu can provide plenty of protein for a power-packed brunch?

Calories **204**	Cholesterol **0mg**	Dietary fiber **4g**
Total fat **9g**	Sodium **81mg**	Sugars **5g**
Saturated fat **1.5g**	Carbohydrates **9g**	Protein **20g**

the INGREDIENTS

1½ cups kale, coarse stalks removed, leaves roughly chopped

1 tsp olive oil

1 green onion, finely chopped

½ cup button mushrooms, quartered

1 cup silken tofu

sea salt and freshly ground black pepper

1 tomato, halved, seeds removed, and flesh chopped

handful of flat-leaf parsley, chopped (plus a few leaves for garnish)

the PREP

1 Steam the kale for 10 minutes, then set aside.

2 Meanwhile, heat the olive oil in a nonstick frying pan on medium heat, then add the green onion and cook for 1 minute. Add the mushrooms and cook for 2 more minutes or until they begin to turn golden brown.

3 Add the silken tofu, stirring it around the pan. Season with salt and pepper and continue stirring until the mixture starts to scramble.

4 Stir in the tomato, parsley, and kale, seasoning with more salt and pepper to taste.

5 Spoon the scrambled tofu mix into a serving bowl, then sprinkle with flat-leaf parsley leaves.

the BUILD

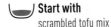 **Start with** scrambled tofu mix

 Add in tomato and kale

 Finish with flat-leaf parsley

Smoked mackerel hash
with harissa yogurt

prep **15 MIN**   cook **25 MIN**

Smoked mackerel is a convenient source of protein and omega-3 fatty acids, handy to have in the fridge.

Calories **562**	Cholesterol **79mg**	Dietary fiber **4g**
Total fat **37g**	Sodium **1,027mg**	Sugars **11g**
Saturated fat **7g**	Carbohydrates **25g**	Protein **31g**

the INGREDIENTS

1 cup Yukon Gold potatoes, peeled and halved

sea salt and freshly ground black pepper

2 radishes, trimmed and sliced

2 tsp rice vinegar

¼ cup beets, cooked and diced

2 tsp olive oil

2 green onions, finely chopped

¼ green chili pepper, seeds removed and finely sliced

4½ oz (125g) smoked mackerel, skinned and roughly flaked

1 tbsp chopped fresh dill

1 tbsp chopped fresh chives

For the dressing

1 tbsp 0% fat plain Greek yogurt

1 tsp harissa

juice of ¼ lemon

the PREP

1 Put the potatoes in a saucepan with enough salted cold water to cover. Cook for 15 minutes, or until tender when pierced with a sharp knife. Drain. As soon as they're cool enough to handle, cut into slices. Set aside.

2 Toss the radishes with 1 tsp of the rice vinegar. Toss the beets with the remaining 1 tsp of rice vinegar and season with salt to taste. Set both aside.

3 Make the dressing by mixing the Greek yogurt, harissa, and lemon juice in a bowl. Season with salt and pepper.

4 Heat the olive oil in a nonstick frying pan on medium heat. Add the potatoes and cook for 2 minutes, then add the green onions and the green chili pepper, stirring for 5 minutes or until the potatoes start to turn golden brown. Add the mackerel and cook for 3 more minutes. Stir in half the dill and chives, then season with pepper.

5 Transfer the mackerel and potato hash to a serving bowl, then add the radishes and beets. Spoon in the yogurt dressing, then sprinkle with the remaining dill and chives.

the BUILD

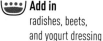 **Start with**
mackerel and
potato hash

 Add in
radishes, beets,
and yogurt dressing

 Finish with
dill and chives

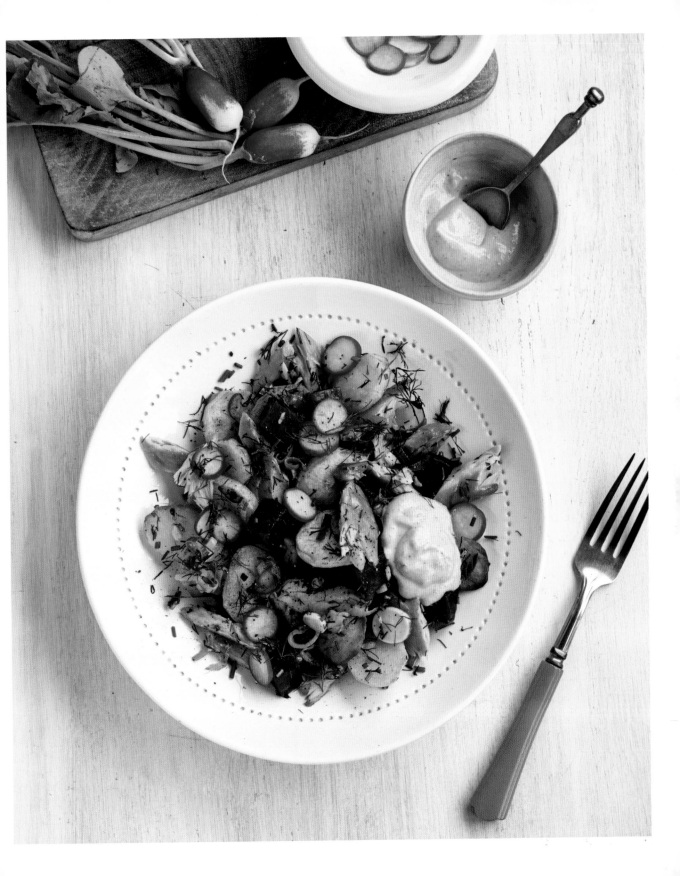

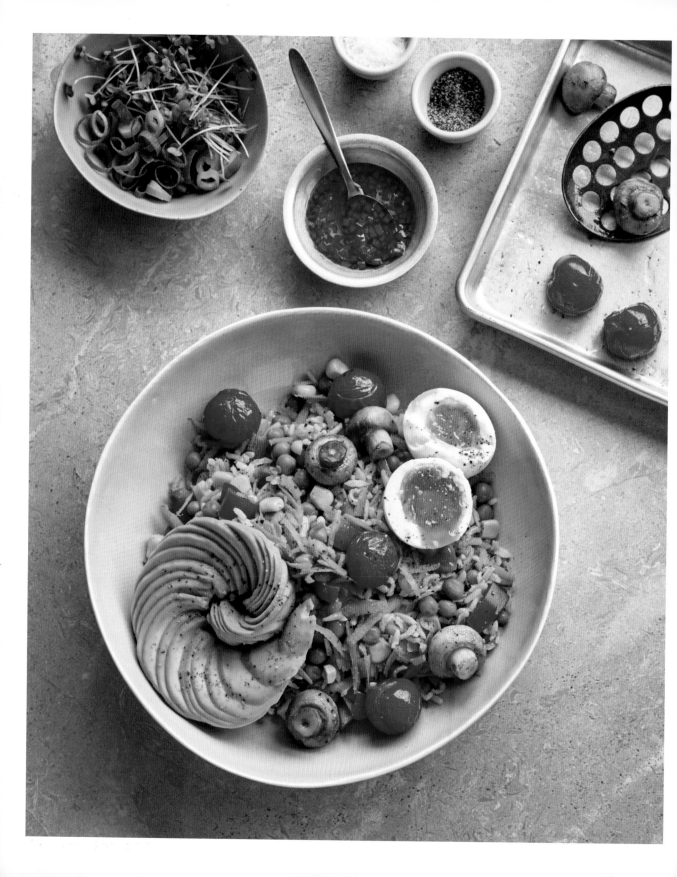

DF   GF   UNDER **600** CALS

Rainbow rice
with chili dressing

prep **15 MIN**   cook **30 MIN**

This brunch will fill you up with protein, and it offers an irresistible array of eye-popping colors.

Calories **500**	Cholesterol **214mg**	Dietary fiber **13g**
Total fat **23g**	Sodium **145mg**	Sugars **12g**
Saturated fat **5g**	Carbohydrates **47g**	Protein **19g**

the INGREDIENTS

⅓ cup brown rice

sea salt and freshly ground black pepper

6 cherry tomatoes

8 button mushrooms

1 tsp olive oil

1 egg

½ cup peas, defrosted if frozen

¼ cup sweet corn

¼ red bell pepper, finely chopped

1 carrot, grated

¼ green chili pepper, finely chopped

½ avocado

1 green onion, green part only, finely sliced

a few cress leaves (optional)

For the dressing

¼ red chili pepper, finely diced

1 tsp rice vinegar

1 tsp mirin rice wine

the PREP

1 Put the brown rice and a pinch of sea salt in a saucepan with ⅔ cup water. Bring to a boil, then reduce the heat to a simmer, cover, and cook for 20–25 minutes or until the rice is tender and the water has been absorbed.

2 Meanwhile, preheat the oven to 400°F (200°C). Mix the tomatoes, mushrooms, and olive oil in a roasting pan, then season with salt and pepper. Roast for 10–15 minutes or until the mushrooms are golden brown.

3 Put the egg into a saucepan with cold water to cover, bring to a boil, and cook for 5 minutes. Drain, plunge into cold water, and, once cool enough to handle, peel and halve it.

4 Add the peas, sweet corn, red bell pepper, carrot, and green chili pepper to the rice. Season with salt and pepper to taste, stir to combine, and set aside.

5 Make the dressing by mixing the red pepper, rice vinegar, and mirin in a bowl, then season with salt and pepper.

6 Spoon the rainbow rice into a serving bowl, then add the egg, tomatoes, and mushrooms. Peel and slice the avocado and place on top. Sprinkle over the green onion and cress leaves, and spoon on the dressing.

the BUILD

 Start with
rainbow rice mixture

 Add in
egg, tomatoes, mushrooms, and avocado

 Finish with
green onion and red chili pepper dressing

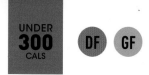
Mexican scrambled eggs
with tomatoes

prep **5 MIN**   cook **10 MIN**

Scrambled eggs are a delicious and filling way to start the day—with chili peppers to wake up your taste buds.

Calories **276**	Cholesterol **427g**	Dietary fiber **9.5g**
Total fat **15.5g**	Sodium **226mg**	Sugars **9g**
Saturated fat **3.5g**	Carbohydrates **10g**	Protein **19.5g**

the INGREDIENTS

2 cups spinach leaves

1 tsp olive oil

1 green onion, finely chopped

½ red chili pepper, finely chopped

½ garlic clove, finely chopped

sea salt and freshly ground black pepper

½ red Romano pepper, finely sliced

2 tomatoes, halved, seeds removed, and flesh chopped

2 eggs, lightly beaten

small handful of cilantro leaves

the PREP

1 Put the spinach leaves in a bowl and cover it with plastic wrap. Microwave the spinach for 1 minute or until it wilts. (Or you can steam it over boiling water for 1 minute.)

2 Heat the olive oil in a nonstick frying pan on medium-high heat, then add the green onion and red chili pepper and cook for 1 minute. Add the garlic, season with salt and pepper, and cook for 1 more minute.

3 Add the red Romano pepper and tomatoes to the pan and stir for 2 minutes, then reduce the heat under the pan to medium-low.

4 Add the beaten eggs to the pan, stirring and folding to combine. Cook for a few more minutes until the eggs begin to scramble.

5 Spoon the scrambled eggs into a serving bowl, then add the spinach and sprinkle with the cilantro leaves.

the BUILD

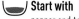 **Start with**
pepper and tomatoes

 add in
eggs and spinach

 Finish with
cilantro leaves

DF — **UNDER 400 CALS**

Nasi goreng
with poached egg

prep **10 MIN**   cook **10 MIN**

This take on Indonesian fried rice is super-tasty, especially when topped with a protein-packed egg.

Calories **310**	Cholesterol **213mg**	Dietary fiber **5.5g**
Total fat **7.5g**	Sodium **404mg**	Sugars **8g**
Saturated fat **1.5g**	Carbohydrates **43g**	Protein **14g**

the INGREDIENTS

1 tsp olive oil

½ small yellow onion, finely chopped

½ garlic clove, finely chopped

sea salt and freshly ground black pepper

1 small carrot, grated

1 cup cooked brown rice

2 cups spinach leaves

1 tsp dark soy sauce

juice of ½ lime

1 egg

1 green onion, green part only, finely sliced

½ red chili pepper, finely chopped

lime wedge (optional)

the PREP

1 Heat the olive oil in a nonstick frying pan on medium-high heat, then add the onion and cook for 1 minute. Add the garlic, season with salt and pepper, and cook for 1 more minute. Add the carrot, stirring for 1 more minute.

2 Stir in the brown rice, then add the spinach leaves, cooking the spinach until it wilts. Add the dark soy sauce and lime juice and cook for 1 more minute.

3 Meanwhile, heat 2 cups of water in a saucepan until it comes to a boil, then reduce the heat to a high simmer. Carefully crack the egg into the water, and poach for 2 minutes or until the yolk turns opaque.

4 Spoon the brown rice mixture into a serving bowl. Use a slotted spoon to remove the egg from the saucepan and place it on the rice. Sprinkle with the green onion and red chili pepper and add the lime wedge (if using), to squeeze over the dish.

the BUILD

 Start with vegetables and brown rice

 Add in poached egg

 Finish with green onion and red chili pepper

No-cook bowls

No cooking is needed for any of the fantastic meals in this chapter. You can enjoy them on the go, thus avoiding the risks of eating out that can so easily compromise your weight loss plan.

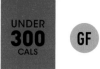

UNDER
300
CALS

GF

Green lentil salad
with feta & pickled red onion

prep **15 MIN**   cook **NONE**

The flavor and color of the pickled red onion contrast beautifully with the nutty lentils and salty feta.

Calories **246**	Cholesterol **28mg**	Dietary fiber **7g**
Total fat **11.5g**	Sodium **635mg**	Sugars **9g**
Saturated fat **5g**	Carbohydrates **17g**	Protein **15g**

the INGREDIENTS

½ cup cooked green lentils

2 tomatoes, halved, seeds removed, and flesh chopped

a few basil leaves, half chopped, the rest left whole

sea salt and freshly ground black pepper

¼ red onion, finely sliced

1 tsp rice vinegar

1 tsp chopped dill

½ cup feta cheese, cubed

¼ cup of pea shoots

1 tbsp pomegranate seeds

For the dressing

2 tsp 0% fat plain Greek yogurt

juice of ¼ lemon

the PREP

1 Mix the green lentils, tomatoes, and chopped basil leaves in a bowl, and season with salt and pepper.

2 Mix the red onion, rice vinegar, and dill in a separate bowl.

3 Make the dressing by mixing the Greek yogurt and lemon juice in a bowl and seasoning with salt and pepper to taste.

4 Spoon the green lentil mixture into a serving bowl, then add the red onion mixture, feta cheese, pea shoots, and pomegranate seeds. Spoon on the yogurt dressing and sprinkle the whole basil leaves over it.

the BUILD

 Start with
green lentil mixture and red onion mixture

 Add in
feta, pea shoots, and pomegranate seeds

 Finish with
yogurt dressing and basil leaves

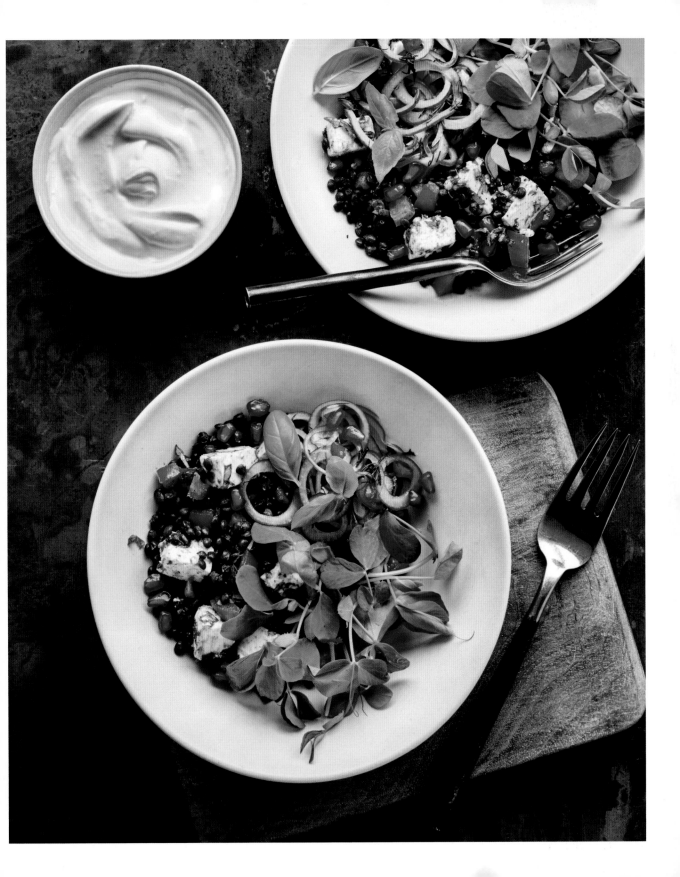

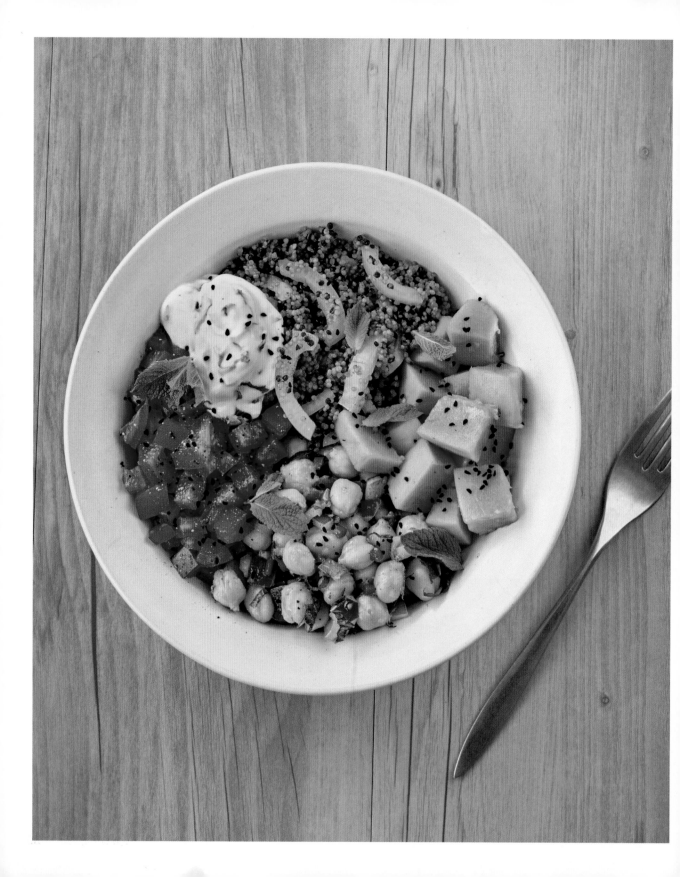

GF

UNDER
600
CALS

Quinoa & chickpeas
with papaya

prep **15 MIN**   cook **NONE**

Indian-inspired spices and chickpeas mingled with tomato and papaya create an explosion of tastes in this bowl.

Calories **521**	Cholesterol **0mg**	Dietary fiber **17g**
Total fat **16g**	Sodium **315mg**	Sugars **20g**
Saturated fat **2g**	Carbohydrates **67g**	Protein **18g**

the INGREDIENTS

½ cup cooked red and white quinoa

¼ yellow pepper, sliced

sea salt and freshly ground black pepper

¾ cup cooked chickpeas

¼ red onion, chopped

¼ red chili pepper, finely chopped

1 in (2.5cm) piece of fresh ginger, peeled and grated

handful of mint leaves, half finely chopped, the rest left whole

1 tbsp 0% fat plain Greek yogurt

2 tomatoes, halved, seeds removed, flesh finely chopped

1 papaya slice, roughly chopped

pinch of nigella seeds

For the dressing

2 tsp olive oil

1 tsp white wine vinegar

¼ tsp medium curry powder

¼ tsp honey

the PREP

1 Mix the quinoa and yellow pepper in a bowl and season with salt and pepper. Set aside.

2 Make the dressing by mixing the olive oil, white wine vinegar, medium curry power, and honey in a bowl, and season with salt and pepper. Set this aside, too.

3 Mix the chickpeas, red onion, red chili pepper, ginger, and half the chopped mint in a bowl. Add the dressing, and season with salt and pepper to taste.

4 Mix the Greek yogurt and remaining chopped mint in a bowl, seasoning with salt to taste.

5 Spoon the quinoa mixture into a serving bowl, then add the chickpeas, tomatoes, and papaya. Spoon on the yogurt mixture, then sprinkle the nigella seeds and the whole mint leaves.

the BUILD

 Start with
quinoa mixture

 Add in
chickpea mixture, tomatoes, and papaya

 Finish with
yogurt mixture, nigella seeds, and mint leaves

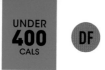

UNDER 400 CALS **DF**

Shrimp & quinoa
with kiwi salsa

prep **10 MIN**   cook **NONE**

Shrimp provides you with protein and zinc, and the kiwi salsa and soy sauce dressing help balance all the flavors.

Calories **341**	Cholesterol **86mg**	Dietary fiber **3g**
Total fat **12g**	Sodium **509mg**	Sugars **12g**
Saturated fat **2g**	Carbohydrates **45g**	Protein **12g**

the INGREDIENTS

4 cherry tomatoes, halved

handful of dill leaves, finely chopped

1 green onion, finely chopped, green and white parts kept separate

sea salt and freshly ground black pepper

½ cup cooked quinoa

½ cup large shrimp, cooked

handful of watercress

pinch of sesame seeds

For the salsa

1 kiwi, finely chopped

1 tsp pomegranate seeds

juice of ½ lime

½ red chili pepper, finely chopped

handful of cilantro leaves, finely chopped

For the dressing

1 tsp extra virgin olive oil

juice of ½ lime

½ tsp dark soy sauce

½ tsp honey

the PREP

1 Mix the cherry tomatoes, dill, and the white part of the green onion in a bowl, and season with salt and pepper.

2 Make the salsa by mixing the kiwi, pomegranate seeds, lime juice, red chili pepper, and cilantro leaves in a bowl, seasoning to taste with salt and pepper. Set aside.

3 Make the dressing by mixing the extra virgin olive oil, lime juice, dark soy sauce, and honey in a bowl, and season with salt and pepper.

4 Spoon the quinoa into a serving bowl, then add the shrimp, watercress, kiwi salsa, and tomato mixture. Sprinkle with the green part of the spring onion and the sesame seeds, and drizzle with the dressing.

the BUILD

 Start with
tomato mixture and kiwi salsa

 Add in
shrimp and watercress

 Finish with
green onion, sesame seeds, and soy sauce dressing

UNDER 600 CALS

Brown rice paella
with tomatoes & shrimp

prep **10 MIN**   cook **NONE**

A take on the classic paella that can be assembled without cooking, making this bowl a filling on-the-go meal.

Calories **428**	Cholesterol **114mg**	Dietary fiber **10g**
Total fat **8g**	Sodium **488mg**	Sugars **10g**
Saturated fat **1g**	Carbohydrates **57g**	Protein **26g**

the INGREDIENTS

¼ cucumber, halved, seeds removed, and sliced

1 green onion, finely chopped

1 tsp rice vinegar

sea salt and freshly ground black pepper

1 cup cooked brown rice

½ cup peas, defrosted if frozen

1 cup sweet corn

2 tomatoes, halved, seeds removed, and flesh chopped

handful of flat-leaf parsley, finely chopped

handful of arugula

85g (3oz) cooked large shrimp

handful of cress (optional)

lemon wedge (optional)

For the dressing

1 tsp extra virgin olive oil

juice of ½ lemon

½ tsp smoked paprika, or 1 tsp regular paprika, plus a little extra to serve

the PREP

1 Make the dressing by whisking the extra virgin olive oil, lemon juice, and smoked paprika in a bowl, seasoning with salt and pepper to taste. Set aside.

2 Mix the cucumber, green onion, and rice vinegar in a bowl, and season with salt and pepper.

3 Spoon the brown rice into a bowl and stir in the peas, sweet corn, and tomatoes, and season with salt and pepper. Add the flat-leaf parsley and lemon dressing and stir again to ensure the rice is coated.

4 Transfer the brown rice and peas mixture to a serving bowl, then add the arugula and shrimp. Spoon in the cucumber mixture, scatter over the cress, and add the lemon wedge for squeezing over (if using). Sprinkle with paprika to serve.

the BUILD

 Start with
brown rice
and peas paella

 Add in
arugula, shrimp, and
cucumber mixture

 Finish with
cress and
lemon wedge

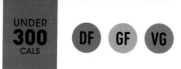

UNDER 300 CALS · DF · GF · VG

Vermicelli rice noodles
with wasabi dressing

prep **15 MIN**   cook **NONE**

There's a real blast of flavor in every mouthful of this dish, thanks to the zingy lime and hot wasabi.

Calories **137**	Cholesterol **0mg**	Dietary fiber **1.5g**
Total fat **5g**	Sodium **12mg**	Sugars **5g**
Saturated fat **0.7g**	Carbohydrates **16g**	Protein **6g**

the INGREDIENTS

1 cup dried vermicelli rice noodles

¾ cup sugar snap peas, finely sliced lengthways

4 radishes, finely sliced

finely grated zest of ½ lime, plus ½ lime, peeled, segmented, and chopped

1 tbsp shelled unsalted pistachios, roughly chopped

a few basil leaves (optional)

handful of cilantro leaves (optional)

lime wedges (optional)

For the dressing

1 cup spinach leaves

3 tbsp silken tofu

1 garlic clove, peeled and halved

juice of ½ lemon

sea salt and freshly ground black pepper

1–2 tsp wasabi, to taste

the PREP

1 Put the vermicelli rice noodles in a bowl and cover with boiling water. Leave for 5 minutes (or according to the package instructions), then drain and set aside.

2 Meanwhile, make the dressing by putting the spinach leaves in a food processor and blending until chopped. Spoon in the silken tofu; add the garlic, lemon juice, and salt and pepper to taste; and blend again. Add the wasabi a little at a time, tasting and adding more wasabi or seasoning as needed, and blend until puréed. Spoon the dressing into a bowl. (This makes 4 servings. Store the extra servings in an airtight container in the fridge for up to 3 days.)

3 Mix the sugar snap peas, radishes, and lime zest in a bowl, season with salt and pepper, then toss with a little of the wasabi dressing.

4 Transfer the noodles to a serving bowl, then add the lime segments. Spoon in the sugar snap peas mixture and the remaining dressing, then sprinkle with the pistachios, basil, and cilantro leaves (if using), and add the lime wedges (if using), to squeeze over the bowl.

the BUILD

 Start with
rice noodles and dressing

 Add in
sugar snap peas mixture and wasabi dressing

 Finish with
pistachios, basil and cilantro leaves, and lime wedges

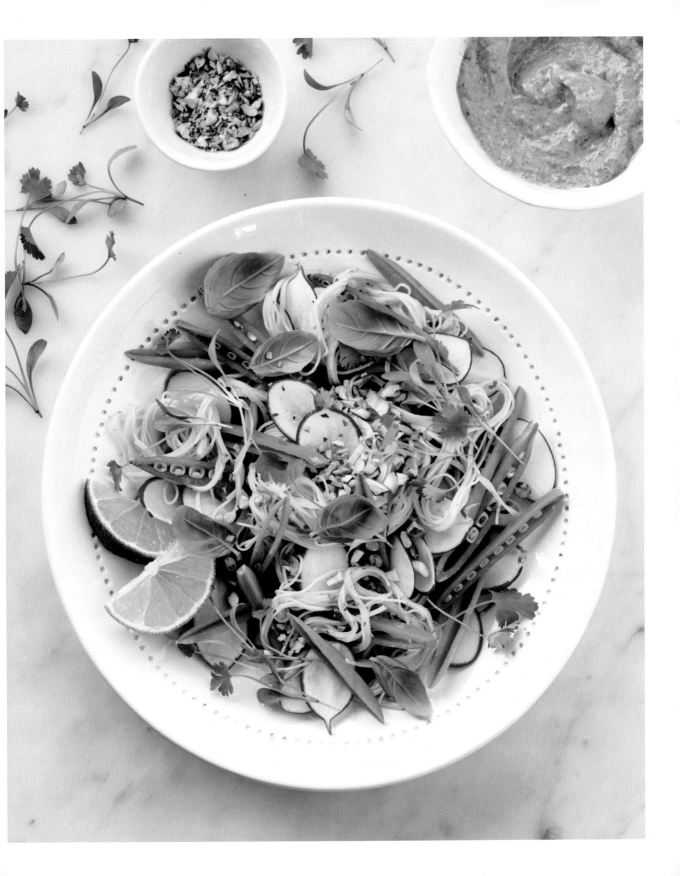

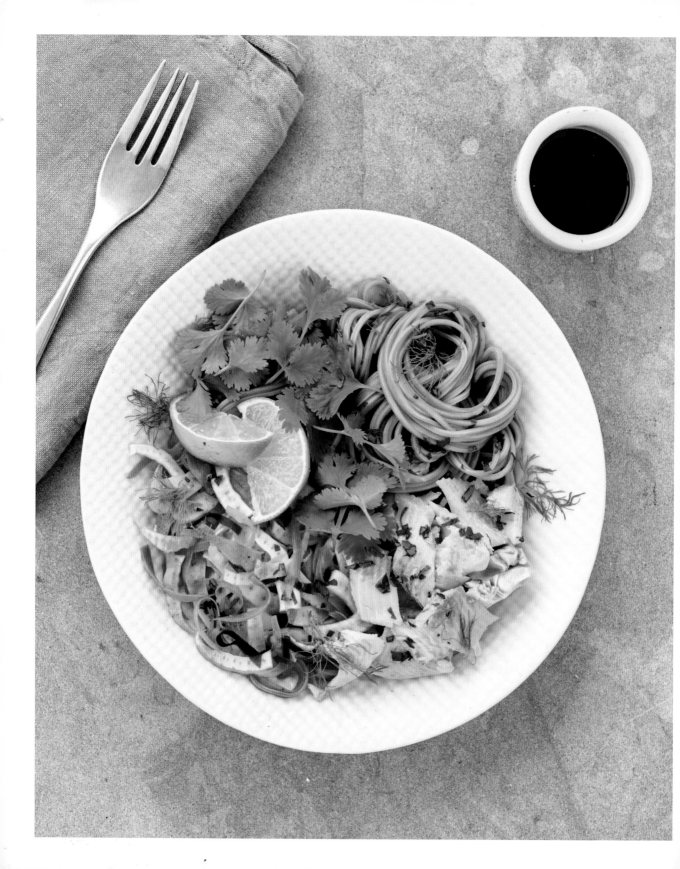

Green tea noodles & trout
with fennel salad

prep **15 MIN**   cook **NONE**

Seaweed brings flavor to this dish without adding calories, making for a fabulously light and delicious meal.

Calories **259**	Cholesterol **21mg**	Dietary fiber **11g**
Total fat **3g**	Sodium **872mg**	Sugars **10.5g**
Saturated fat **0.7g**	Carbohydrates **36g**	Protein **15g**

the INGREDIENTS

1 cup green tea soba noodles

3 pieces of dried wakame

¾ cup fennel, trimmed and finely sliced (reserve fronds for garnish)

½ cup carrot, grated

3½oz (100g) smoked trout, roughly flaked

handful of cilantro leaves, half chopped, the rest left whole

lime slices (optional)

handful of flat-leaf parsley, chopped

For the dressing

1 tsp dark soy sauce

1 tsp mirin rice wine

½ tsp honey

juice of ¼ lime

sea salt and freshly ground black pepper

the PREP

1 Put the green tea soba noodles in a bowl and cover with boiling water. Let them soak for 3–6 minutes (or according to the package instructions), then drain, rinse with cold water to separate, and set aside.

2 Put the wakame in a bowl and cover with boiling water. Leave for 10 minutes or until reconstituted, then drain, and chop roughly.

3 Make the dressing by mixing the dark soy sauce, mirin, honey, and lime juice in a bowl, and season with salt and pepper.

4 Toss the fennel, carrot, and wakame in a bowl, add most of the dressing, and toss again.

5 Put the noodles in a serving bowl, then add the fennel and carrot salad, trout, cilantro leaves, and lime slices (if using) to squeeze over the bowl. Drizzle over the remaining dressing and add the flat-leaf parsley and fennel fronds (if using).

the BUILD

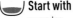 **Start with**
green tea
soba noodles

 Add in
fennel and carrot
salad, trout, cilantro
leaves, and lime slices

 Finish with
soy sauce dressing,
flat-leaf parsley,
and fennel fronds

Smoked salmon sushi
with wasabi dressing

prep **5 MIN**   cook **NONE**

This captures all the tastes of sushi, but it's quick to put together, and brown rice is a healthy addition.

Calories **300**	Cholesterol **9mg**	Dietary fiber **5.5g**
Total fat **16g**	Sodium **259mg**	Sugars **4.5g**
Saturated fat **3.5g**	Carbohydrates **25g**	Protein **10g**

the INGREDIENTS

½ cup cooked brown rice

1 tsp rice vinegar

1½oz (40g) smoked salmon

⅓ cup cucumber, cut into matchsticks

3 radishes, finely sliced

1 green onion, finely sliced

¼ red bell pepper, finely sliced

handful of spinach leaves

½ small avocado

1 tsp pickled ginger

1 tsp sesame seeds

For the dressing

1 tsp rice vinegar

¼ tsp wasabi

sea salt and freshly ground black pepper

the PREP

1 Put the brown rice in a bowl, stir in the rice vinegar, and set aside.

2 Make the dressing by mixing the rice vinegar and wasabi in a bowl and seasoning with salt and pepper.

3 Put the smoked salmon in a serving bowl, then add the cucumber, radishes, green onion, red bell pepper, and spinach leaves. Peel and chop the avocado and scatter it over with the pickled ginger, drizzle over the dressing, and sprinkle with the sesame seeds.

the BUILD

 Start with
smoked salmon

 Add in
cucumber, radishes, green onion, red pepper, and spinach

 Finish with
avocado, ginger, rice vinegar dressing, and sesame seeds

DF **GF** **UNDER 600 CALS**

Carrot & cucumber noodles
with almonds

prep **15 MIN**   cook **NONE**

If you have a spiralizer or mandolin slicer, you can rustle up this nutritious, tasty bowl super-fast.

Calories **500**	Cholesterol **0mg**	Dietary fiber **12g**
Total fat **23g**	Sodium **72mg**	Sugars **23g**
Saturated fat **2g**	Carbohydrates **56g**	Protein **12g**

the INGREDIENTS

2 carrots, peeled and sliced into thin lengths (or use a spiralizer or mandolin slicer)

½ cucumber, seeds removed, and flesh cut into batons

½ red bell pepper, sliced

1 cup bean sprouts

2-in (5cm) piece of fresh ginger, peeled and finely sliced

½ cup cooked white and red quinoa mix

1 tsp rice vinegar

sea salt and freshly ground black pepper

pinch of red pepper flakes

handful of cilantro leaves, chopped

10 almonds, chopped

For the dressing

1 tsp rice vinegar

juice of ½ lime

¼ red chili pepper, finely chopped

¼ tsp honey

the PREP

1 Make the dressing by mixing the rice vinegar, lime juice, red chili pepper, and honey in a bowl, then season with salt and pepper to taste.

2 Put the carrots, cucumber, red bell pepper, bean sprouts, ginger, and dressing in a bowl, then toss with your hands.

3 Mix the white and red quinoa and rice vinegar in a bowl, and season with salt and pepper.

4 Transfer the quinoa mixture to a serving bowl, then add the vegetable noodles. Sprinkle over the red pepper flakes, cilantro leaves, and almonds.

the BUILD

 Start with quinoa and vegetable noodles

 Add in red pepper flakes

 Finish with cilantro leaves and almonds

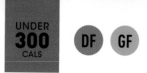

UNDER **300** CALS   DF   GF

Smoked trout & watermelon
with ginger dressing

prep **15 MIN**   cook **NONE**

This is a refreshing and tangy bowl: cool watermelon cuts through the smoked trout's delicate flavor.

Calories **204**	Cholesterol **0mg**	Dietary fiber **2.5g**
Total fat **10g**	Sodium **502mg**	Sugars **8.5g**
Saturated fat **2g**	Carbohydrates **11g**	Protein **16g**

the INGREDIENTS

handful of lamb's lettuce leaves

1 green onion, finely chopped

⅛ cup sugar snap peas, finely sliced

handful of chives, finely chopped

1 tbsp frozen edamame beans, defrosted

1¾oz (50g) smoked trout, flaked

¾ cup watermelon, chopped

pinch of black sesame seeds (optional)

lime wedge (optional)

For the dressing

2 tsp extra virgin olive oil

juice of ¼ lime

1-in (2.5cm) piece of fresh ginger, peeled and grated

1 garlic clove, grated

¼ tsp honey

pinch of paprika

sea salt and freshly ground black pepper

the PREP

1 Make the dressing by mixing the extra virgin olive oil, lime juice, ginger, garlic, honey, and paprika in a bowl, then season with salt and pepper.

2 Toss the lamb's lettuce leaves, green onion, sugar snap peas, chives, and edamame with the dressing.

3 Transfer the salad mixture to a serving bowl, then add the trout and watermelon. Sprinkle over the black sesame seeds (if using) and add the lime wedge (if you wish), to squeeze over the bowl.

the BUILD

 Start with salad mixture and dressing

 Add in trout and watermelon

 Finish with black sesame seeds and lime wedge

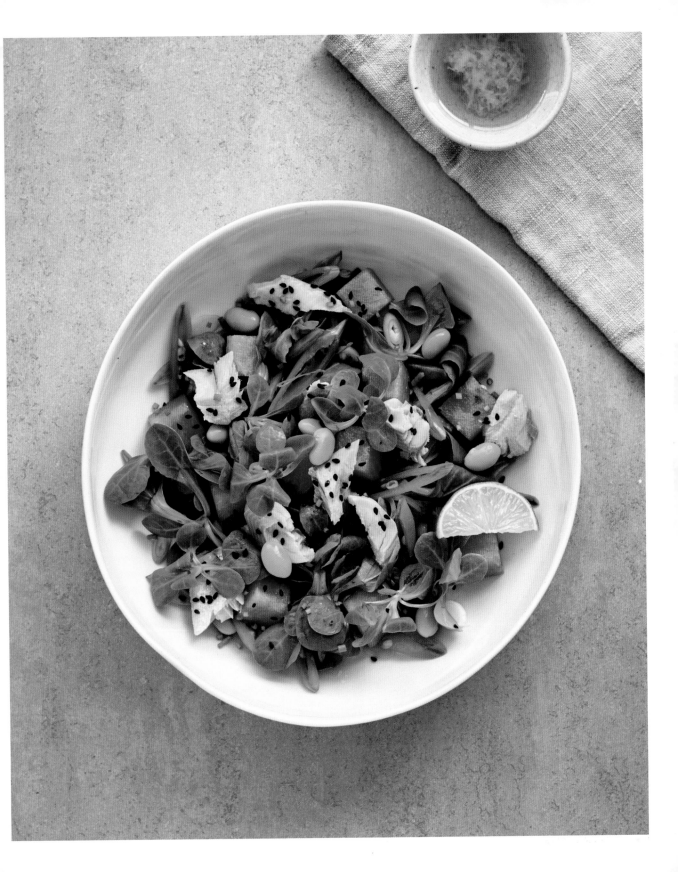

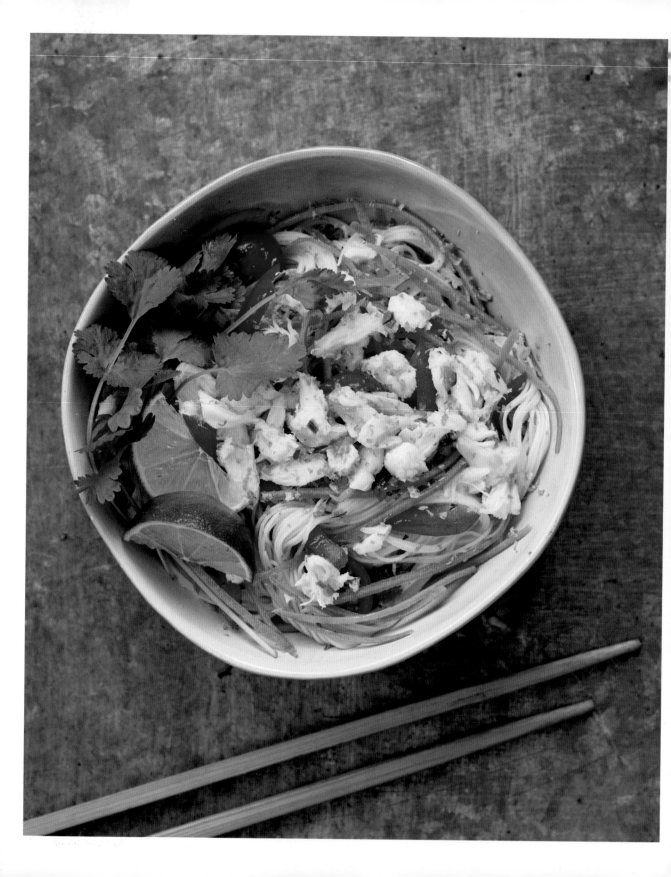

DF GF

UNDER
300
CALS

Vermicelli noodles & crab
with jalapeño & honey dressing

prep **10 MIN**   cook **NONE**

An excellent source of omega-3 fatty acids, crab is also low in calories, so it's perfect for a tasty weight loss bowl.

Calories **295**	Cholesterol **33mg**	Dietary fiber **5g**
Total fat **11g**	Sodium **195mg**	Sugars **8.5g**
Saturated fat **1.5g**	Carbohydrates **30g**	Protein **17g**

the INGREDIENTS

1 cup dried vermicelli rice noodles

½ cup carrot, cut into fine strips

¼ red bell pepper, cut into fine strips

5 cherry tomatoes, halved

sea salt and freshly ground black pepper

handful of cilantro leaves

½ cup fresh white crabmeat

finely grated zest of ¼ lime

4 almonds, roughly chopped

lime wedges (optional)

For the dressing

2 tsp extra virgin olive oil

¼ jalapeño pepper, finely chopped

juice of ¼ lime

¼ tsp honey

the PREP

1 Put the vermicelli noodles in a bowl and cover with boiling water. Leave for 5 minutes (or according to the package instructions), then drain, and set aside.

2 Once the noodles have cooled, mix them with the carrot, red bell pepper, and tomatoes. Season with salt and pepper, then stir in half the cilantro leaves.

3 Make the dressing by mixing the extra virgin olive oil, jalapeño pepper, lime juice, and honey in a small bowl, then season with salt and pepper.

4 Toss the noodle mix with half the dressing and transfer to a serving bowl, then add the crab, lime zest, the remaining cilantro leaves, and almonds. Drizzle over the remaining dressing and add lime wedges (if using), to squeeze over the bowl.

the BUILD

 Start with
vermicelli noodle mixture

 Add in
crab, lime zest, cilantro leaves, and almonds

 Finish with
jalapeño and honey dressing and lime wedges

Salmon & bean sprouts
with cucumber relish & mango

prep **10 MIN**   cook **NONE**

Rich salmon matches well with sweet mango and cool cucumber for a light and healthy bowl packed with flavor.

Calories **473**	Cholesterol **101mg**	Dietary fiber **4.5g**
Total fat **19.5g**	Sodium **1,196mg**	Sugars **15.5g**
Saturated fat **4g**	Carbohydrates **34g**	Protein **38g**

the INGREDIENTS

5oz (140g) hot-smoked salmon fillet, skinned and roughly flaked

handful of arugula

½ cup cooked red and white quinoa mix

handful of bean sprouts

½ cup mango, finely chopped

pinch of finely ground pink peppercorns, or freshly ground black pepper

a few mint leaves

For the relish

½ cup cucumber, finely chopped

¼ red bell pepper, finely chopped

¼ red chili pepper, finely chopped

1 tsp rice vinegar

¼ small red onion, finely chopped

sea salt and freshly ground black pepper

For the dressing

1 tsp extra virgin olive oil

1 tsp rice vinegar

juice of ½ lime

¼ tsp honey

the PREP

1 Make the relish by mixing the cucumber, red bell pepper, red chili pepper, rice vinegar, and red onion in a bowl, and season with salt and pepper to taste. Set aside.

2 Make the dressing by whisking the extra virgin olive oil, rice vinegar, lime juice, and honey in a bowl, and season this, too, with salt and pepper to taste.

3 Put the salmon in a serving bowl, then add the arugula, red and white quinoa, bean sprouts, and mango. Spoon over the cucumber relish, drizzle with the dressing, then sprinkle over the ground pink peppercorns and mint leaves.

the BUILD

 Start with
cucumber relish

 Add in
salmon, arugula, quinoa, bean sprouts, and mango relish

 Finish with
cucumber relish, dressing, pink peppercorns, and mint leaves

DF GF **UNDER 400 CALS**

Brown rice, crabmeat & fennel
with pink grapefruit

prep **10 MIN**   cook **NONE**

This low-calorie bowl really fills you up with protein-rich crab and rice, and is given a zing from citrus fruits.

Calories **309**	Cholesterol **26.5mg**	Dietary fiber **6.5g**
Total fat **2.5g**	Sodium **180mg**	Sugars **12.5g**
Saturated fat **0.5g**	Carbohydrates **53g**	Protein **16g**

the INGREDIENTS

⅓ cup fresh white crabmeat

1 green onion, finely chopped

¼ cucumber, halved, seeds removed, and sliced

pinch of red pepper flakes

sea salt and freshly ground black pepper

1 grapefruit, peeled and segmented (reserve juice)

½ cup cooked brown rice

½ cup fennel, finely sliced, and tossed in lemon juice (reserve fronds for garnish)

5 radishes, finely sliced

handful of watercress

the PREP

1   Mix the crab, green onion, cucumber, and red pepper flakes in a bowl, then season with some salt and pepper. Add the reserved grapefruit juice, and stir again.

2   Spoon the brown rice into a serving bowl, then add the crabmeat mixture, fennel, radishes, and watercress. Finish with the grapefruit segments.

the BUILD

 Start with brown rice

 Add in crabmeat mixture, fennel, radishes, and watercress

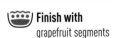 **Finish with** grapefruit segments

UNDER
400
CALS

GF

Chicken & black-eyed peas
with spicy yogurt dressing

prep **15 MIN**   cook **NONE**

This bowl offers a spicy hot sauce kick, but soothing black-eyed peas and vibrant citrus provide contrast.

Calories **399**	Cholesterol **102mg**	Dietary fiber **14g**
Total fat **5.5g**	Sodium **110mg**	Sugars **10g**
Saturated fat **1.5g**	Carbohydrates **29g**	Protein **51g**

the INGREDIENTS

1 cup cooked black-eyed peas

finely grated zest of 1 lemon

½ jalapeño, finely chopped

pinch of cumin seeds, crushed

sea salt and freshly ground black pepper

¼ red bell pepper, finely chopped

1 tomato, halved, seeds removed, and flesh finely chopped

1 celery stalk, finely chopped

¼ red onion, finely sliced

1 tbsp pomegranate seeds

pinch of sumac

a few cilantro leaves

4½ oz (125g) cooked skinless chicken breast, sliced

4 Little Gem lettuce leaves

finely grated lime zest, to serve (optional)

For the dressing

2 tbsp 0% fat plain Greek yogurt

a few drops of hot sauce

the PREP

1 Mix the black-eyed peas, lemon zest, jalapeño, and cumin seeds in a bowl, and season with salt and pepper. Stir in the red bell pepper, tomato, and celery, then check the seasoning, adding more as needed.

2 Mix the red onion, pomegranate seeds, sumac, and cilantro leaves in another bowl, seasoning with salt and pepper to taste.

3 Make the dressing by mixing the Greek yogurt and hot sauce in a bowl. Season with salt and pepper to taste.

4 Put the black-eyed peas mixture and the chicken into a serving bowl, then add the Little Gem lettuce. Spoon on the red onion mixture and spicy yogurt dressing and squeeze over the lime zest (if using).

the BUILD

 Start with
black-eyed peas mixture and chicken

 Add in
Little Gem lettuce

 Finish with
red onion mixture, spicy yogurt dressing, and lime zest

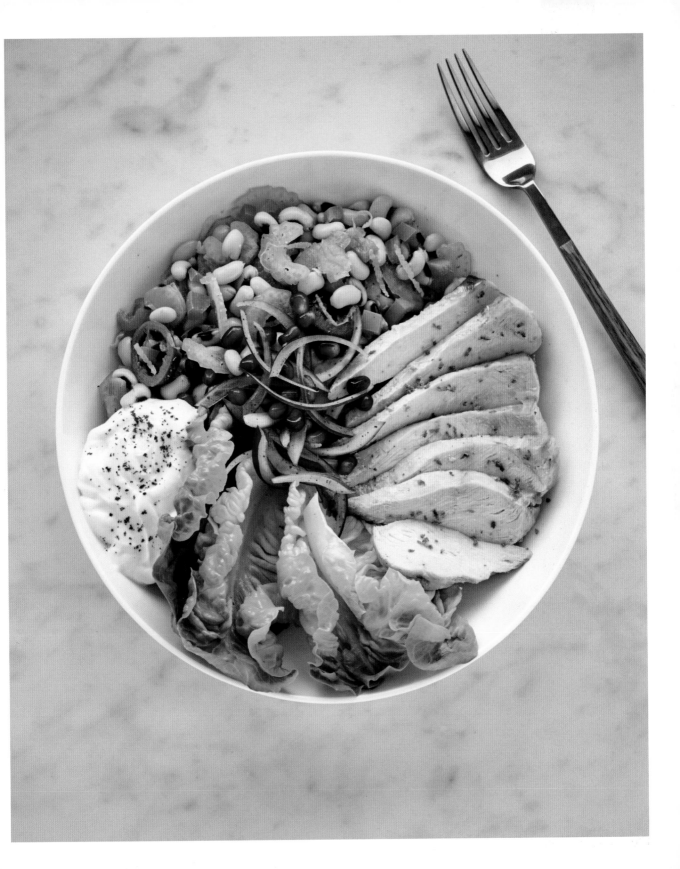

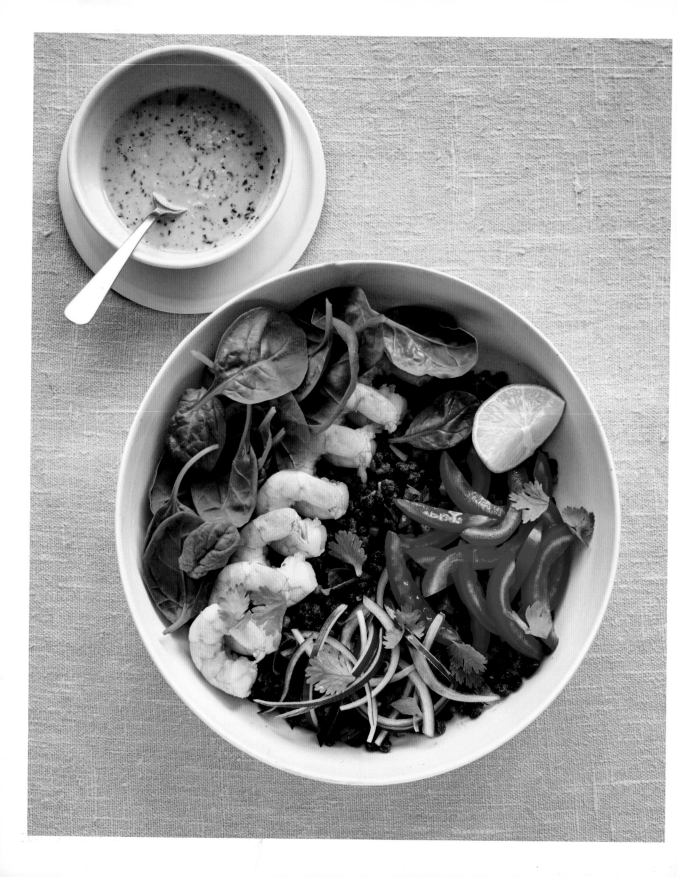

UNDER 400 CALS

Shrimp & curried lentils
with herbed cashew dressing

prep **15 MIN**   cook **NONE**

This flavor-packed bowl has a spicy taste as well as a sweet dressing, while shrimp is great for protein.

Calories **333**	Cholesterol **73g**	Dietary fiber **11g**
Total fat **7.5g**	Sodium **314mg**	Sugars **7.5g**
Saturated fat **1.5g**	Carbohydrates **35g**	Protein **26g**

the INGREDIENTS

1 cup cooked green lentils

½ tsp ground turmeric

1-in (2.5cm) piece of fresh ginger, peeled and grated or finely chopped

¼ red chili pepper, finely chopped

¼ tsp extra virgin olive oil

handful of cilantro leaves, half chopped, the rest left whole

sea salt and freshly ground black pepper

½ cup cooked large shrimp

handful of spinach leaves

1 tomato, halved, seeds removed, and flesh sliced

¼ cup red onion, finely sliced

lime wedge (optional)

For the dressing

¼ cup cashews

handful of cilantro leaves

pinch of red pepper flakes

juice of ¼ lime

¼ tsp honey

the PREP

1 Mix the green lentils, turmeric, ginger, red chili pepper, extra virgin olive oil, and chopped cilantro leaves in a bowl. Season with salt and pepper to taste, and set aside.

2 Make the dressing by blending the cashews in a food processor until finely chopped. Add 4 tbsp of water, the cilantro leaves, red pepper flakes, lime juice, and honey, and season with salt and pepper. Blend again until mixed, but retaining some texture. (This makes 2 portions. Store the extra portion in an airtight container in the fridge for up to 3 days.)

3 Spoon the green lentil mixture into a serving bowl, then add the shrimp, spinach, tomato, and red onion. Spoon on the dressing, sprinkle with the whole cilantro leaves, and add the lime wedge (if using), to squeeze over.

the BUILD

 Start with
green lentil mixture

 Add in
shrimp, spinach, tomato, and red onion

 Finish with
cashew dressing, cilantro leaves, and lime wedge

Chicken & sugar snap peas
with red chili dressing

prep **10 MIN**   cook **NONE**

A bowl with many complex flavor profiles—spicy, sweet, sour, and umami—ideal in an all-in-one salad.

Calories **464**	Cholesterol **103mg**	Dietary fiber **7g**
Total fat **6g**	Sodium **93mg**	Sugars **13g**
Saturated fat **1.5g**	Carbohydrates **49g**	Protein **50g**

the INGREDIENTS

1½oz (40g) vermicelli rice noodles

1 cup bean sprouts

1 green onion, finely chopped

¼ red onion, finely chopped

1 cup sugar snap peas, finely sliced on the diagonal

¼ papaya, finely sliced

¼ cucumber, sliced into fine batons

handful of cilantro leaves, finely chopped

4½ oz (125g) cooked skinless chicken breast, shredded

a few mint leaves

pinch of red pepper flakes (optional)

lime wedge (optional)

For the dressing

juice of ½ lime

1 tsp rice vinegar

¼ red chili pepper, finely chopped

sea salt and freshly ground black pepper

the PREP

1 Add the vermicelli rice noodles to a bowl and cover with boiling water. Leave for 5 minutes (or according to the package instructions), then drain, rinse, and drain again. Return them to the bowl.

2 Make the dressing by mixing the lime juice, rice vinegar, and red chili pepper in a bowl, then season with salt and pepper.

3 Mix the bean sprouts, green onion, red onion, sugar snap peas, papaya, cucumber, and cilantro leaves in a bowl with your hands, and season with salt and pepper. Add the dressing and half the chicken and mix again.

4 Transfer the noodles to a serving bowl, then add the remaining chicken and the vegetable mixture. Sprinkle with the mint leaves and red pepper flakes (if using) and add the lime wedge (if using), to squeeze over the bowl.

the BUILD

 Start with
vermicelli rice noodles, chicken, and vegetable mixture

 Add in
mint leaves and red pepper flakes

 Finish with
lime wedge

Wheatberries & papaya
with lime pickle relish

prep **10 MIN**   cook **NONE**

There's an exotic Indian aroma to this bowl, thanks to the spicy lime pickle and the cool tamarind yogurt.

Calories **365**	Cholesterol **0mg**	Dietary fiber **12g**
Total fat **9g**	Sodium **396mg**	Sugars **17.5g**
Saturated fat **1g**	Carbohydrates **53g**	Protein **12g**

the INGREDIENTS

1 tbsp 0% fat plain Greek yogurt

½ tsp tamarind paste

1 carrot, grated

pinch of nigella seeds

1 tsp rice vinegar

sea salt and freshly ground black pepper

½ red bell pepper, finely chopped

handful of mint leaves, finely chopped

juice of ½ lime

1 cup cooked quinoa, lentils, and wheatberries mix

handful of spinach leaves

¼ papaya, sliced

lime wedge (optional)

For the relish

1 lime, peeled and segmented

¼ red chili pepper, finely chopped

¼ red onion, finely sliced

the PREP

1 Mix the Greek yogurt and tamarind paste in a bowl and set aside.

2 Toss the carrot, nigella seeds, and rice vinegar in a bowl, and season with salt and pepper. Set aside.

3 Stir the red pepper, mint, and lime juice into the quinoa, lentils, and wheatberries mix, and season with salt and pepper to taste.

4 Make the relish by mixing the lime, red chili pepper, and red onion in a bowl, and season with salt and pepper.

5 Spoon the wheatberries mixture into a serving bowl, then add the carrot mixture, lime pickle relish, spinach leaves, and papaya. Spoon on the tamarind yogurt and add the lime wedge (if using), to squeeze over.

the BUILD

 Start with
wheatberries mixture

 Add in
carrot mixture, lime pickle relish, spinach leaves, and papaya

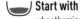 **Finish with**
tamarind yogurt and lime wedge

Vegan sushi Buddha bowl
with nori

prep **15 MIN**   cook **NONE**

This bowl's diverse textures and tastes provide plenty of vital nutrients and lots of different vegetables to enjoy.

Calories **420**	Cholesterol **0mg**	Dietary fiber **11g**
Total fat **12g**	Sodium **60mg**	Sugars **9g**
Saturated fat **2g**	Carbohydrates **53g**	Protein **19g**

the INGREDIENTS

¾ cup cooked brown rice

3 tsp rice vinegar

1 sheet of dried nori, finely cut into strips with scissors

2 tsp black sesame seeds

1-in (2.5cm) piece of fresh ginger, peeled and grated

½ cup frozen edamame, defrosted

½ cup carrot, sliced into thick sticks

⅓ cup firm tofu, cut into cubes

½ cup cucumber, sliced into half-moon shapes

1 green onion, white part only, sliced lengthwise

3 radishes, trimmed and finely sliced

½ cup sugar snap peas, finely sliced

handful of chives, finely chopped

handful of red amaranth leaves (optional)

½ tsp wasabi paste

the PREP

1 Mix the brown rice, 1½ tsp of the rice vinegar, the nori, and 1 tsp of the black sesame seeds in a bowl. Set aside.

2 Mix the ginger and the remaining 1½ tsp of rice vinegar in a separate bowl.

3 Transfer the rice mixture to a serving bowl, then arrange over the edamame, carrot, tofu, cucumber, green onion, radishes, sugar snap peas, chives, and red amaranth (if using) in groups. Spoon on the wasabi paste, or serve it on the side, then sprinkle over the ginger mixture and the remaining black sesame seeds.

the BUILD

 Start with
rice, edamame, carrot, tofu, cucumber, and green onion

 Add in
chives, radishes, sugar snap peas, and red amaranth

Finish with
wasabi paste, ginger mixture, and black sesame seeds

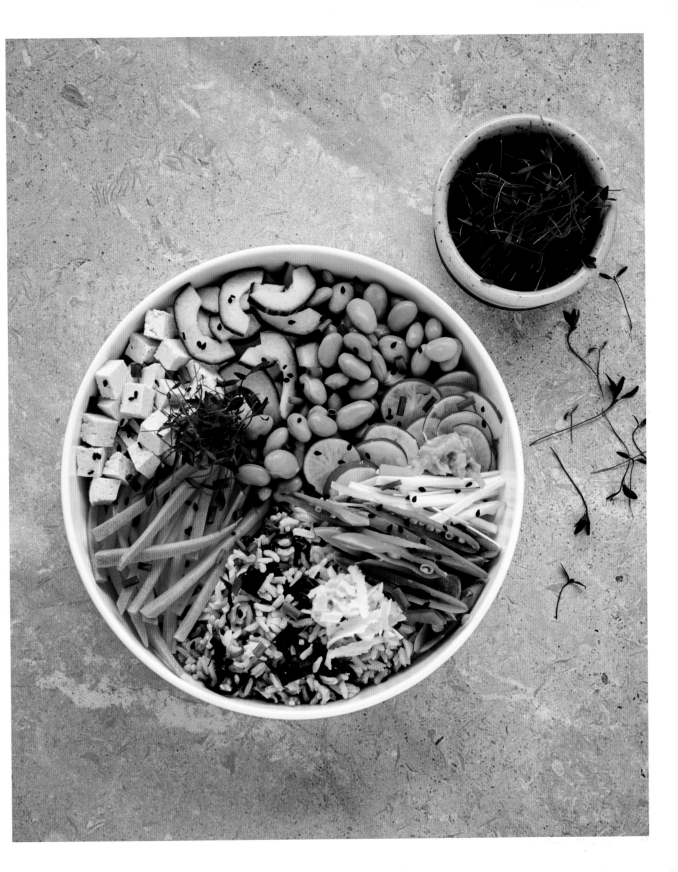

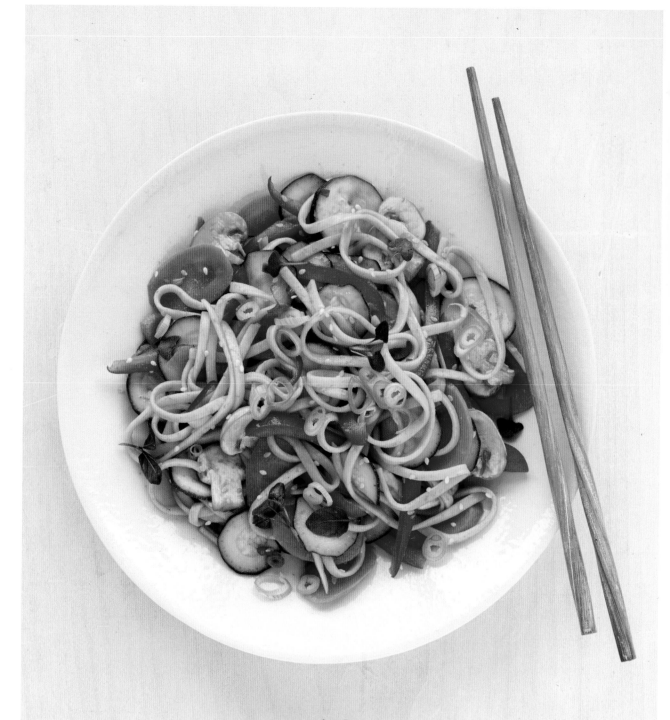

No-cook veggie stir-fry
with rice vinegar

prep **20 MIN**   cook **NONE**

You can make this bowl quickly, and all the vegetables need is the tangy dressing to bring out their sweetness.

Calories **293**	Cholesterol **0mg**	Dietary fiber **7g**
Total fat **7g**	Sodium **300mg**	Sugars **10g**
Saturated fat **1.5g**	Carbohydrates **44g**	Protein **11g**

the INGREDIENTS

1 cup flat rice noodles

1 cup carrot, finely sliced

1 cup zucchini, finely sliced

½ red bell pepper, finely sliced

¼ red chili pepper, finely sliced

2 tsp sesame seeds

1-in (2.5cm) piece of lemongrass, outer leaves removed, inner part finely sliced

½ cup button mushrooms, halved

1 green onion, trimmed, green part finely sliced, and white part sliced lengthwise

a few purple basil leaves (optional)

For the dressing

1 tsp dark soy sauce

1 tsp rice vinegar

juice of ½ lime

½ garlic clove, grated

¼ red chili pepper, finely chopped

sea salt and freshly ground black pepper

the PREP

1   Put the rice noodles in a bowl and cover with boiling water. Leave for 10 minutes (or according to the package instructions), then drain and set aside.

2   Make the dressing by mixing the dark soy sauce, rice vinegar, lime juice, garlic, and red chili pepper in a bowl, and season with salt and pepper to taste.

3   Combine the carrot, zucchini, red bell pepper, red chili pepper, sesame seeds, lemongrass, mushrooms, and the white part of the green onion in a bowl. Add half the noodles and season with salt and pepper. Mix, trickle in the rice vinegar dressing, and mix again.

4   Transfer the no-cook stir-fry mix to a serving bowl, then add the remaining noodles. Sprinkle over the green part of the green onion and the purple basil leaves (if using).

the BUILD

 Start with
no-cook veggie
stir-fry mixture

 Add in
rice noodles and
rice vinegar dressing

 Finish with
green onion and
purple basil leaves

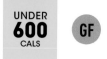

Lentils, mint & blueberries
with beets

prep **10 MIN**   cook **NONE**

Blueberries might seem an unusual pairing with lentils, but their tartness enhances the nutty legumes.

Calories **418**	Cholesterol **14mg**	Dietary fiber **21g**
Total fat **7g**	Sodium **696mg**	Sugars **12.5g**
Saturated fat **3g**	Carbohydrates **49g**	Protein **29g**

the INGREDIENTS

1 cup frozen baby or regular fava beans

1 cooked beet, chopped

5 radishes, trimmed and sliced

1 cup cooked green lentils

handful of mint leaves, finely chopped

½ cup cucumber, peeled, seeds removed, and chopped

½ cup blueberries

handful of wild arugula

¼ cup feta cheese, finely chopped (optional)

For the dressing

juice of ½ lime

pinch of paprika

sea salt and freshly ground black pepper

the PREP

1 Put the beans in a bowl and cover with boiling water. Leave for 5 minutes, or until tender, then drain. (You can peel them now, if you prefer.) Once cooled, toss them with the beet and radishes. Set aside.

2 Make the dressing by mixing the lime juice and paprika in a bowl and season with salt and pepper to taste.

3 Mix the green lentils, mint leaves, cucumber, and blueberries in a bowl, and season with salt and pepper.

4 Spoon the green lentils mixture into a serving bowl, then add the beans mixture and arugula. Sprinkle with the feta (if using) and drizzle over the lime dressing.

the BUILD

 Start with
green lentils mixture

 Add in
fava beans mixture and arugula

 Finish with
feta and lime dressing

DF GF

UNDER 600 CALS

Rainbow coleslaw
with wasabi & trout

prep **10 MIN**   cook **NONE**

This rainbow coleslaw is an excellent addition to rich trout, and the wasabi dressing pulls it all together.

Calories **417**	Cholesterol **0mg**	Dietary fiber **12g**
Total fat **10.5g**	Sodium **619mg**	Sugars **23g**
Saturated fat **2g**	Carbohydrates **51g**	Protein **24g**

the INGREDIENTS

½ cup cooked red and white quinoa mix

2oz (60g) smoked trout fillet

handful of watercress

pinch of chia seeds

3 radishes, sliced into matchsticks

For the coleslaw

1 cup red cabbage, shredded

1 medium carrot, grated

1 Gala apple, halved, cored, and finely sliced

sea salt and freshly ground black pepper

For the dressing

1 tsp extra virgin olive oil

1 tsp apple cider vinegar

½-in (1.5cm) piece of fresh ginger, peeled and grated

½ tsp wasabi paste

the PREP

1   Make the coleslaw by mixing the red cabbage, carrot, and apple in a bowl, and season with salt and pepper to taste. Set aside. (This makes 2 portions. Store the extra portion in an airtight container in the fridge for up to 3 days.)

2   Make the dressing by whisking the extra virgin olive oil, cider vinegar, ginger, and wasabi paste in a bowl, and season with salt and pepper to taste. Pour the dressing over the coleslaw and mix well together.

3   Spoon the quinoa mix into a serving bowl, then add the rainbow coleslaw, flake in the trout, add the watercress, and scatter over the chia seeds and radish matchsticks.

the BUILD

 Start with
quinoa mix

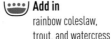 **Add in**
rainbow coleslaw, trout, and watercress

 Finish with
chia seeds and radishes

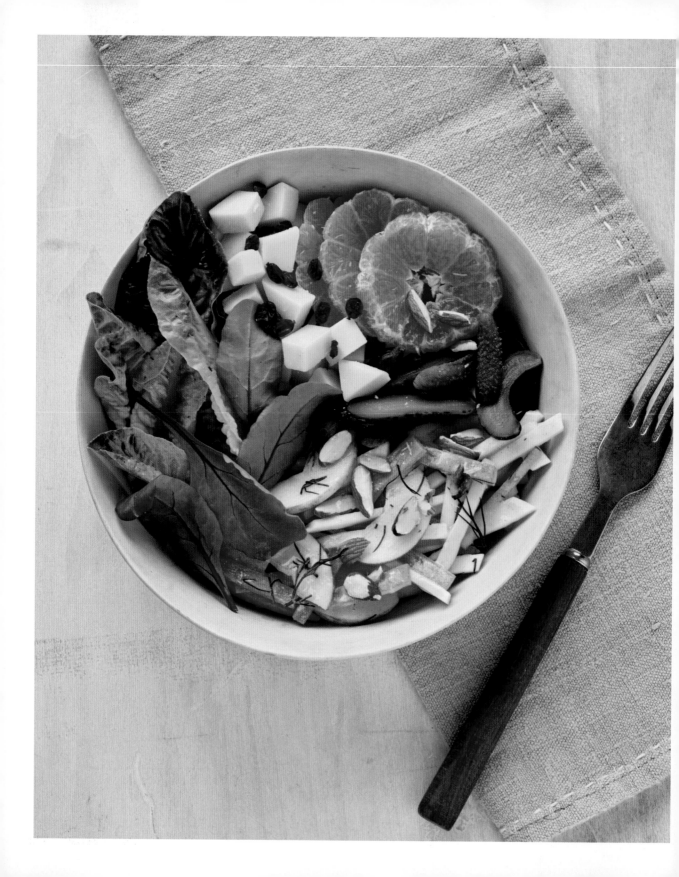

Sour celeriac coleslaw
with almonds & Edam

prep **15 MIN**   cook **NONE**

A coleslaw without mayonnaise has fewer calories, but can have just as much taste if you add a mellow cheese.

Calories **218**	Cholesterol **14mg**	Dietary fiber **5g**
Total fat **11.5g**	Sodium **281mg**	Sugars **15.5g**
Saturated fat **4g**	Carbohydrates **16g**	Protein **10g**

the INGREDIENTS

1 cup celeriac

juice of 1 lemon

1 tsp barberries

½ cup carrot, finely sliced

½ Gala apple, finely sliced

sea salt and freshly ground black pepper

1 tsp white wine vinegar

¼ tsp Dijon mustard

1 tsp chopped dill

⅓ cup Edam cheese, cut into cubes (or use another low-fat cheese)

1 gherkin (sweet pickle), finely sliced

handful of mixed salad leaves

1 clementine, peeled and sliced

6 skin-on almonds, chopped

the PREP

1 Finely slice the celeriac into batons, then toss with the lemon juice, to prevent discoloration.

2 Put the barberries in a small bowl, cover with water, and leave to soak for 10 minutes, then drain.

3 Mix the celeriac, carrot, and apple in a bowl, and season with salt and pepper to taste, then stir in the white wine vinegar, Dijon mustard, and dill.

4 Spoon the sour coleslaw into a serving bowl, then add the Edam, gherkin, salad leaves, and clementine. Scatter over the almonds and barberries.

the BUILD

 Start with
sour coleslaw

 Add in
Edam, gherkin,
salad leaves,
and clementine

 Finish with
almonds
and barberries

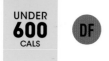

UNDER 600 CALS · **DF**

Soba noodles & mackerel
with pink pepper & beets

prep **15 MIN**   cook **NONE**

A bowl full of superfoods thanks to the beets, nori, and mackerel—all given a vibrant tang from the dressing.

Calories **548**	Cholesterol **47mg**	Dietary fiber **4.5g**
Total fat **23g**	Sodium **932mg**	Sugars **6.5g**
Saturated fat **4g**	Carbohydrates **50g**	Protein **32g**

the INGREDIENTS

1 cup soba noodles

2½ oz (75g) smoked mackerel, skinned and flaked

1 cup cucumber, sliced into matchsticks

handful of cilantro leaves, chopped

½ cup frozen edamame, defrosted

¼ sheet nori, cut into fine strips

½ cup raw or vacuum-packed pickled beets, grated

1 green onion, green part only, finely sliced

freshly ground pink peppercorns

For the dressing

1 tsp rice vinegar

1-in (2.5cm) piece of fresh ginger, peeled and grated

¼ garlic clove, grated

juice of ¼ lime

handful of cilantro leaves, chopped

pinch of red pepper flakes

sea salt and freshly ground black pepper

the PREP

1 Put the soba noodles in a bowl and cover with boiling water. Leave for 10 minutes (or according to the package instructions), then drain, rinse with cold water to separate, drain again, and set aside.

2 Make the dressing by mixing the rice vinegar, ginger, garlic, lime juice, cilantro leaves, and red pepper flakes in a bowl, seasoning with salt and pepper.

3 Toss the smoked mackerel, cucumber, and cilantro leaves with the noodles, add the dressing, and toss again.

4 Transfer the noodle and mackerel mix to a serving bowl, then add the edamame and nori. Spoon in the beets, and scatter over the green onion and pink pepper.

the BUILD

 Start with
noodle and mackerel mixture

 Add in
edamame, nori, and beets

 Finish with
green onion and pink peppercorns

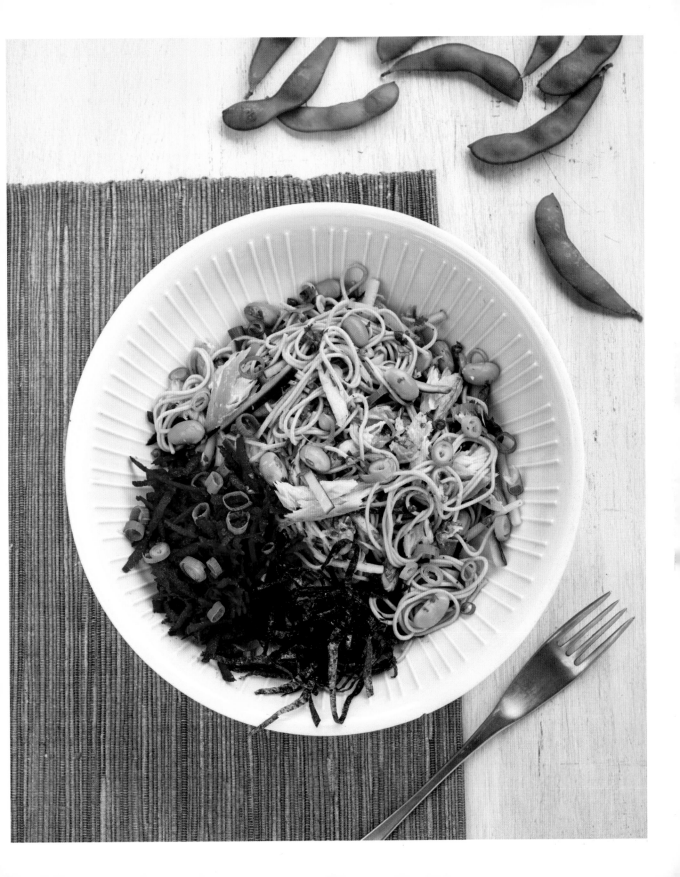

Vegan brown rice sushi
with miso & soy

prep **5 MIN**   cook **NONE**

This bowl is deconstructed sushi, giving you all the deliciousness you expect without the fuss.

Calories **421**	Cholesterol **0mg**	Dietary fiber **10g**
Total fat **23g**	Sodium **505**mg	Sugars **7g**
Saturated fat **5g**	Carbohydrates **40g**	Protein **10g**

the INGREDIENTS

1 cup cooked brown rice

1 tsp rice vinegar

½ sheet nori, finely chopped

½ cup red cabbage, shredded

1 carrot, grated

3 radishes, finely sliced

½ avocado

½ tsp black sesame seeds

½ tsp white sesame seeds

lime wedge (optional)

For the dressing

1 tsp rice vinegar

1 tsp dark soy sauce

1 tsp barley miso

½ tsp white sesame seeds

½ tsp black sesame seeds

sea salt and freshly ground black pepper

the PREP

1 Put the brown rice in a bowl, stir in the rice vinegar and nori, and set aside.

2 Make the dressing by whisking the rice vinegar, dark soy sauce, barley miso, white sesame seeds, and black sesame seeds in a bowl, seasoning with salt and pepper.

3 Spoon the brown rice mixture into a serving bowl, then add the red cabbage, carrot, and radishes, and chop in the avocado. Sprinkle over the black and white sesame seeds, drizzle with the miso dressing, and add the lime wedge (if using) to squeeze over the bowl.

the BUILD

 Start with
brown rice mixture, red cabbage, carrot, radishes, and avocado

 Add in
sesame seeds and miso dressing

 Finish with
lime wedge

Brown rice & sashimi tuna
with watermelon

prep **10 MIN**   cook **NONE**

Essentially a poke (*poh-kay*) full of umami: tangy tuna and salty nori served with sweet watermelon.

Calories **358**	Cholesterol **35mg**	Dietary fiber **5g**
Total fat **3g**	Sodium **376mg**	Sugars **13.5g**
Saturated fat **0.5g**	Carbohydrates **50g**	Protein **30.5g**

the INGREDIENTS

3½oz (100g) sashimi-grade tuna, cut into bite-sized chunks

1 tsp dark soy sauce

1 green onion, finely sliced, green and white parts kept separate

pinch of sesame seeds

freshly ground black pepper

1 cup cooked brown rice

½ sheet nori, finely sliced

1 tsp rice vinegar

1 carrot, grated

½ cup watermelon, cut into cubes

4 radishes, finely sliced

1 tsp pickled ginger

the PREP

1 Put the tuna in a bowl, then stir in the dark soy sauce, the white part of the green onion, the sesame seeds, and the pepper. Set aside.

2 Put the brown rice in another bowl, and stir in the nori and rice vinegar.

3 Spoon the brown rice mixture into a bowl, then add the tuna mixture, carrot, watermelon, and radishes. Sprinkle with the green part of the green onion and add the pickled ginger.

the BUILD

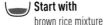 **Start with**
brown rice mixture

 Add in
tuna mixture, carrot, watermelon, and radishes

 Finish with
green onion and pickled ginger

Speedy
bowls

These recipes don't take long to prep and cook—all of them can be made within 30 minutes—but they'll keep you satisfied. They are also huge on flavor, but not loaded with calories.

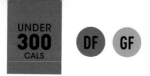

UNDER 300 CALS · **DF** · **GF**

Squid, carrot & cucumber
with saffron dressing

prep **15 MIN**   cook **5 MIN**

Squid is an excellent and delicious low-calorie fast food that works well in this spicy, crunchy, tangy bowl.

Calories **200**	Cholesterol **225mg**	Dietary fiber **4.5g**
Total fat **9g**	Sodium **157mg**	Sugars **7.5g**
Saturated fat **1.5g**	Carbohydrates **8.5g**	Protein **19g**

the INGREDIENTS

5½ oz (150g) baby squid, cleaned, washed, and cut into rings (including tentacles)

2 tsp extra virgin olive oil

pinch of red pepper flakes, plus extra to serve

sea salt and freshly ground black pepper

1 cup cucumber, peeled into ribbons with a vegetable peeler

1 cup carrot, peeled into ribbons with a vegetable peeler

½ cup bean sprouts

1 celery stalk, trimmed and sliced at an angle

2 tsp pomegranate seeds

½ green onion, green part only, finely chopped

lime wedge (optional)

For the dressing

pinch of saffron threads

2½ tsp white wine vinegar

the PREP

1 Mix the squid, extra virgin olive oil, and red pepper flakes in a bowl, and season with salt and pepper. Heat a griddle pan on high heat, then add the squid mixture, cooking for 90 seconds on each side or until the squid begins to turn golden brown. (Be careful not to overcook the squid, or it will become rubbery.) Set aside.

2 Make the dressing by putting the saffron threads in a bowl and adding a little hot (but not boiling) water. (Too much saffron will be overpowering, and boiling water makes the spice less effective.) Leave until cool, then mix in the white wine vinegar and season with salt and pepper.

3 Toss the cucumber and carrot ribbons with a little of the saffron dressing.

4 Put the squid mixture in a serving bowl, then add the cucumber and carrot ribbons, bean sprouts, celery, and pomegranate seeds. Drizzle with the remaining dressing, sprinkle with red pepper flakes and green onion, and add the lime wedge (if using) to squeeze over the bowl.

the BUILD

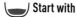 **Start with**
squid mixture, cucumber, and carrot

 Add in
bean sprouts, celery, and pomegranate seeds

 Finish with
saffron dressing, red pepper flakes, green onion, and lime wedge

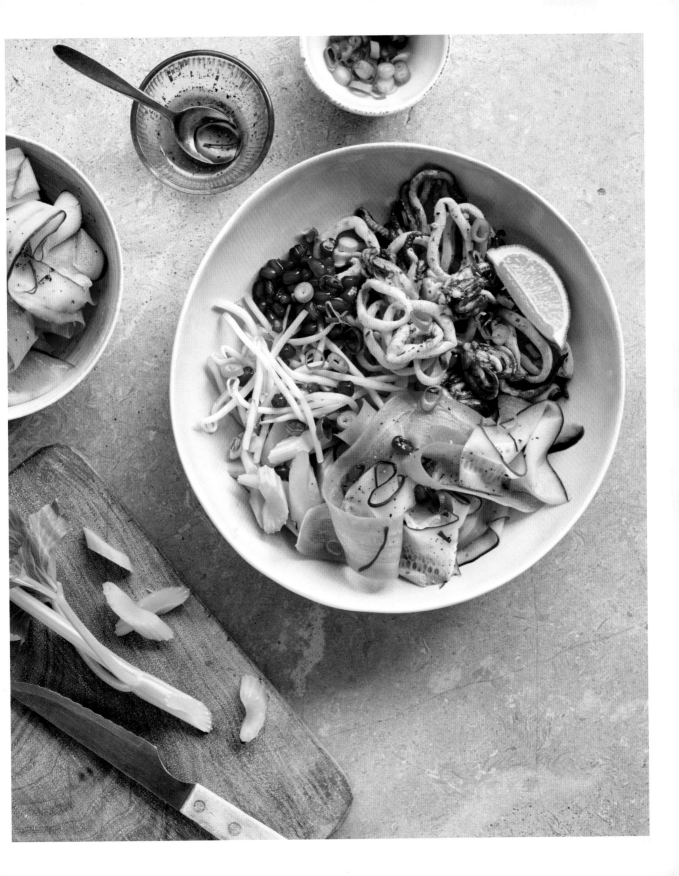

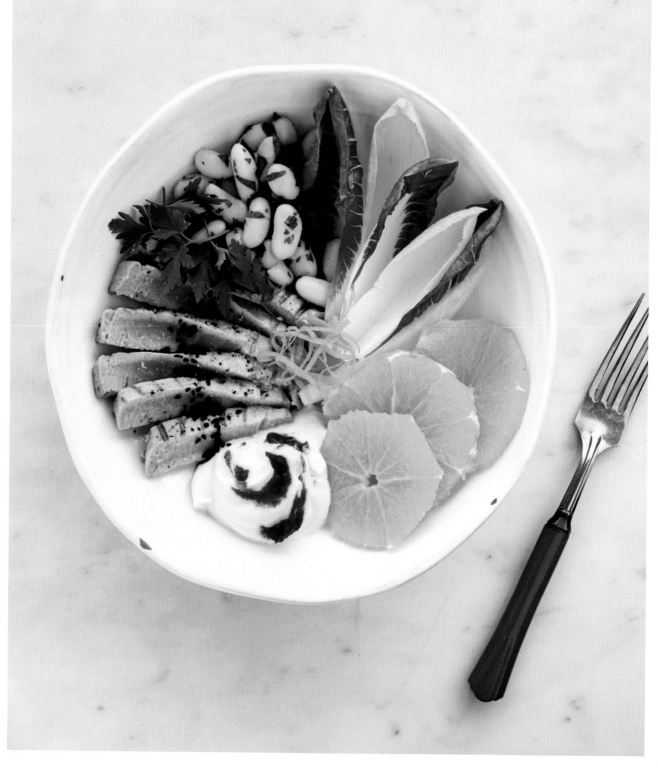

GF · UNDER **300** CALS

Tuna steak & cannellini
with chicory & citrus

prep **5 MIN**   cook **10 MIN**

This bowl might be low on calories but scores high on flavor and nutrition; ideal for a quick meal at any time.

Calories **256**	Cholesterol **35mg**	Dietary fiber **5.5g**
Total fat **8g**	Sodium **469mg**	Sugars **3.5g**
Saturated fat **1g**	Carbohydrates **13g**	Protein **31g**

the INGREDIENTS

3½ oz (100g) tuna steak

2 tsp extra virgin olive oil

sea salt and freshly ground black pepper

¼ cup cooked cannellini beans

2 tsp lemon juice

1 tbsp finely chopped flat-leaf parsley

5 red or white chicory leaves

3 orange slices

pinch of nigella seeds

For the dressing

2 tsp 0% fat plain Greek yogurt

finely grated zest of 1 orange

½ tsp harissa (optional)

the PREP

1 Coat the tuna steak with 1 tsp of the extra virgin olive oil and season with salt and pepper. Heat a griddle pan over a high heat, put in the tuna, and cook for 2–3 minutes on each side, leaving it a little pink in the middle. Allow to rest for at least 5 minutes.

2 Mix the cannellini beans, lemon juice, flat-leaf parsley, and the remaining 1 tsp of extra virgin olive oil in a bowl, then season with salt and pepper. Set aside.

3 Make the dressing by mixing the Greek yogurt, orange zest, and harissa (if using) in a bowl. Alternatively, mix the yogurt and orange zest, and swirl over the harissa.

4 Slice the tuna across the grain and put it in a serving bowl, then add the cannellini bean mixture, chicory leaves, and orange slices. Spoon on the citrus dressing and sprinkle over the nigella seeds.

the BUILD

 Start with
tuna steak

 Add in
cannellini beans, chicory leaves, and orange slices

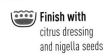 **Finish with**
citrus dressing and nigella seeds

Gazpacho salad
with hot sauce dressing

prep **15 MIN**   cook **15 MIN**

This has all the ingredients of a classic gazpacho soup, but is served as a colorful, sweet, and tasty salad.

Calories **583**	Cholesterol **3.4mg**	Dietary fiber **14g**
Total fat **28g**	Sodium **43mg**	Sugars **15g**
Saturated fat **4.5g**	Carbohydrates **44g**	Protein **32g**

the INGREDIENTS

2 tomatoes, quartered

1 tsp olive oil

pinch of ground cinnamon

pinch of red pepper flakes

sea salt and freshly ground black pepper

½ cup cooked beets, roughly chopped

½ cup cucumber, sliced into half-moon shapes

¼ red bell pepper, roughly chopped

¼ green bell pepper, roughly chopped

1 celery stick, trimmed and sliced

1 garlic clove, grated

1 green onion, green part only, finely sliced

½ avocado

juice of 1 lemon

a few basil leaves

For the dressing

1 tsp extra virgin olive oil

a few drops of hot sauce

the PREP

1 Preheat the oven to 400°F (200°C). Mix the tomatoes, olive oil, cinnamon, and red pepper flakes in a roasting pan, and season with salt and pepper. Roast for 10–15 minutes, or until the tomatoes start to split. Set aside.

2 Mix the beets, cucumber, red bell pepper, green bell pepper, celery, garlic, and green onion in a bowl.

3 Make the dressing by mixing the extra virgin olive oil and hot sauce in a bowl, then toss it with the vegetables, add the roasted tomatoes, and toss again.

4 Chop the avocado roughly, then toss with the lemon juice to prevent discoloration.

5 Spoon the gazpacho salad into a serving bowl, then add the avocado and sprinkle the basil leaves over the salad.

the BUILD

 Start with gazpacho salad

 Add in avocado

 Finish with basil leaves

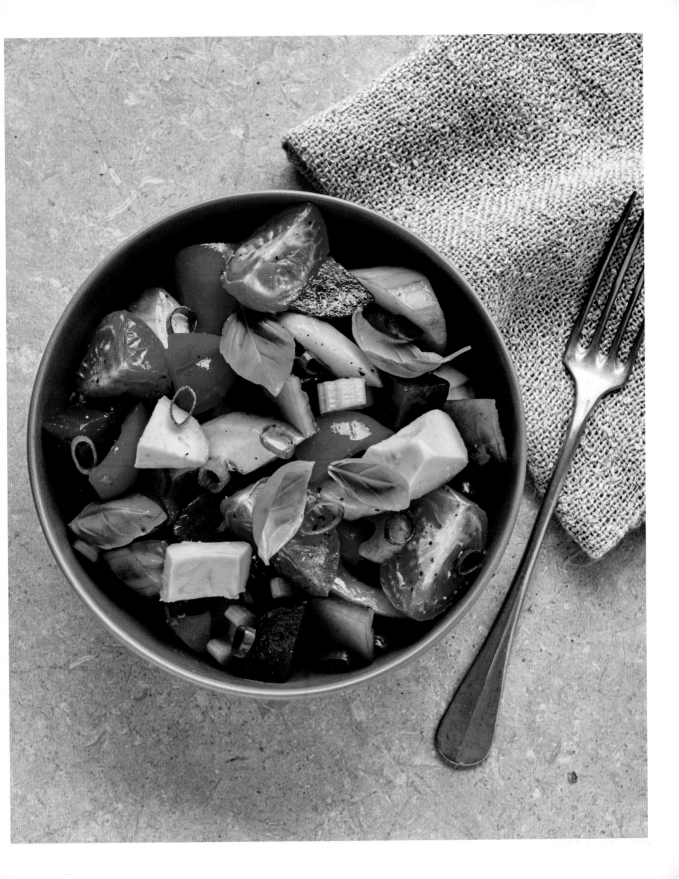

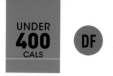

UNDER 400 CALS · DF

Bulgur wheat & tomatoes
with tahini & chickpeas

prep **10 MIN**   cook **15 MIN**

Bulgur wheat provides plenty of fiber for your daily needs, while the tahini gives this bowl a great nuttiness.

Calories **341**	Cholesterol **0mg**	Dietary fiber **14g**
Total fat **11.5g**	Sodium **52mg**	Sugars **15g**
Saturated fat **2g**	Carbohydrates **40g**	Protein **12g**

the INGREDIENTS

1 cup bulgur wheat

sea salt and freshly ground black pepper

¼ red onion, finely chopped

handful of dill, finely chopped

2 tomatoes, halved, seeds removed, and flesh finely chopped

1 tsp extra virgin olive oil

handful of flat-leaf parsley, finely chopped

⅓ cup cooked chickpeas

juice of ½ lemon

1 carrot, peeled into ribbons with a vegetable peeler

handful of mint leaves, chopped

1 tsp rice vinegar

1 green onion, finely chopped

handful of watercress

For the dressing

1 tsp extra virgin olive oil

1 tsp white wine vinegar

1 tsp tahini paste

½ tsp honey

the PREP

1   Put the bulgur wheat and a pinch of sea salt in a saucepan with 2 cups of water. Cover and cook for 10–15 minutes, topping it off with hot water if needed. Allow to cool, keeping the lid on, for 5 minutes.

2   Mix the red onion, dill, tomatoes, extra virgin olive oil, and flat-leaf parsley into the bulgur, then season generously with salt and pepper.

3   Make the dressing by whisking the extra virgin olive oil, white wine vinegar, tahini paste, and honey in a bowl, and season with salt and pepper to taste.

4   Mix the chickpeas, lemon juice, and plenty of freshly ground black pepper in a separate bowl.

5   Mix the carrot, mint leaves, rice vinegar, green onion, and salt and pepper in another separate bowl.

6   Fluff up the bulgur wheat with a fork and transfer it to a serving bowl, then add the watercress, chickpea mixture, and carrot mixture. Spoon on the tahini dressing.

the BUILD

 Start with
bulgur wheat

 Add in
watercress, chickpea mixture, and carrot mixture

 Finish with
tahini dressing

UNDER 600 CALS

Squash & chipotle beans
with baked egg

prep **10 MIN**   cook **20 MIN**

This hot, spicy dish is the very definition of comfort food, but takes little effort to make.

Calories **425**	Cholesterol **213mg**	Dietary fiber **11g**
Total fat **10.5g**	Sodium **118mg**	Sugars **9g**
Saturated fat **2g**	Carbohydrates **54g**	Protein **23g**

the INGREDIENTS

1 chipotle chili pepper

1 cup butternut squash, peeled, and roughly chopped

¼ red bell pepper, roughly chopped

1 tsp olive oil

sea salt and freshly ground black pepper

6 cherry tomatoes

1 green onion, roughly chopped

1 tsp apple cider vinegar

1 cup cooked black-eyed peas, pinto beans, or a mixture

½ cup cooked brown rice

1 egg

1 cup spinach leaves

a few cilantro leaves (optional)

the PREP

1 Preheat the oven to 400°F (200°C). Put the chipotle chili pepper in a large cup, cover with warm water, and leave to soak for 10 minutes, then drain.

2 Mix the butternut squash, red bell pepper, and olive oil in a roasting pan, seasoning with salt and pepper. Roast for 15 minutes, or until the squash is tender. Set aside.

3 Blend the cherry tomatoes, green onion, apple cider vinegar, and chipotle chili pepper in a food processor. Pour the mixture into a saucepan, season with salt and pepper, and heat on low for 5–10 minutes. Stir in the black-eyed peas, pinto beans, or a mixture of both.

4 Spoon the beans into an ovenproof dish or frying pan, then add the brown rice, roasted squash, and red bell pepper. Crack the egg over the mixture, put a lid on the bowl or pan, and put it in the oven for 3 minutes, or until the egg has cooked.

5 Transfer to a serving bowl, then add the spinach and sprinkle with the cilantro leaves (if using).

the BUILD

 Start with
squash, beans, and egg mixture

 Add in
spinach leaves

 Finish with
cilantro leaves

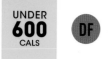
Smoked mackerel & cabbage
with orange & miso

prep **10 MIN**   cook **20 MIN**

Mackerel and orange are a fantastic pairing, also offering omega-3 fatty acids and vitamin C.

Calories **491**	Cholesterol **19mg**	Dietary fiber **6g**
Total fat **20g**	Sodium **425mg**	Sugars **11g**
Saturated fat **3.5g**	Carbohydrates **59g**	Protein **16g**

the INGREDIENTS

½ cup red Camargue and wild rice mix

1 cup red cabbage, finely shredded

handful of cilantro leaves, chopped, plus a few whole leaves for garnish

1 cup bean sprouts

½ sheet nori, finely sliced

1½ oz (40g) smoked mackerel, skinned and flaked

½ orange, peeled and segmented

For the dressing

1 tsp extra virgin olive oil

juice of ½ orange

2½ in (6.5cm) piece of fresh ginger, peeled and finely sliced or grated

sea salt and freshly ground black pepper

1 tsp barley miso

the PREP

1 Put the rice in a saucepan with 2 cups of water. Bring to a boil, then reduce the heat to a gentle simmer, cover, and cook for 15–20 minutes, or according to the package instructions, until the rice is tender and the water has been absorbed. Set aside, keeping the lid on.

2 Make the dressing by mixing the extra virgin olive oil, orange juice, and ginger in a bowl, and season with salt and pepper to taste. Remove and reserve half the dressing and mix the barley miso into the other half. Taste the miso dressing and adjust the seasoning with salt and pepper.

3 Mix the shredded red cabbage with half the chopped cilantro leaves and the reserved orange dressing.

4 Toss the cooked rice with the remaining chopped cilantro leaves and spoon it into a serving bowl, then add the bean sprouts, nori, red cabbage mixture, mackerel, and orange segments. Drizzle over the orange and miso dressing and scatter the whole cilantro leaves on top.

the BUILD

 Start with
red Camargue and wild rice mix

 Add in
bean sprouts, nori, cabbage mixture, mackerel, and orange

 Finish with
orange and miso dressing and cilantro leaves

DF **GF** **UNDER 600 CALS**

Kale & poached salmon
with red pepper salsa

prep **15 MIN**   cook **15 MIN**

This bowl delivers lots of power nutrients, from dark green kale and red bell pepper to oily fish and almonds.

Calories **500**	Cholesterol **84mg**	Dietary fiber **7g**
Total fat **25g**	Sodium **267mg**	Sugars **3g**
Saturated fat **4g**	Carbohydrates **33g**	Protein **33g**

the INGREDIENTS

1 tsp flaked almonds

4½ oz (125g) salmon fillet, skinned

2 cups kale, coarse stems removed, leaves chopped

1 cup cooked quinoa and whole-grain rice mix

pinch of paprika

For the salsa

⅓ cup red bell pepper, finely chopped

¼ cucumber, seeds removed and flesh finely chopped

1 green onion, finely chopped, white and green parts kept separate

½ garlic clove, finely chopped or grated

pinch of paprika

2 tsp red wine vinegar

sea salt and freshly ground black pepper

the PREP

1 Spoon the flaked almonds into a small dry frying pan, place on medium heat, and cook, stirring, until they turn a shade darker and smell toasted. Remove to a plate.

2 Put the salmon in a medium-sized frying pan and cover it with water. Put a lid on the pan and simmer gently for 10 minutes or until the salmon becomes tender and opaque. Remove it carefully with a spatula. When the salmon is cool enough to handle, flake it into chunky pieces, and set aside.

3 Make the salsa by mixing the red bell pepper, cucumber, white part of the green onion, garlic, paprika, and red wine vinegar in a bowl, then season with salt and pepper.

4 Meanwhile, steam the kale for 10 minutes or until tender. (Don't overcook the kale; you want to retain as many nutrients as possible.)

5 Spoon the quinoa and whole-grain rice mix into a serving bowl, then add the kale and salmon. Spoon in the red bell pepper salsa and sprinkle over the reserved green part of the green onion, the toasted almonds, and the paprika.

the BUILD

 Start with
quinoa and whole-grain rice mix, kale, and salmon

 Add in
red bell pepper salsa

 Finish with
green onion, almonds, and paprika

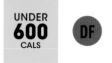

UNDER **600** CALS DF

Herbed turkey tabbouleh
with pistachios

prep **10 MIN**   cook **10 MIN**

This bowl of lean turkey and nutty bulgur is enlivened by herbs, lemony sumac, and sweet pomegranate.

Calories **466**	Cholesterol **57mg**	Dietary fiber **9g**
Total fat **16g**	Sodium **133mg**	Sugars **3g**
Saturated fat **2.5g**	Carbohydrates **37g**	Protein **38g**

the INGREDIENTS

3½ oz (100g) turkey breast

1 tsp olive oil

sea salt and freshly ground black pepper

1 cup cooked bulgur wheat

handful of flat-leaf parsley, finely chopped

handful of mint leaves, finely chopped

handful of dill, finely chopped

2 tsp pomegranate seeds

pinch of sumac

juice of ½ lemon

handful of spinach leaves

10 pistachios, finely chopped

½ tsp harissa

the PREP

1 Brush the turkey breast with the olive oil, then season with some salt and pepper. Heat a griddle pan on high, then add the turkey, cooking it for 2–3 minutes or until it easily comes away from the pan. Flip it over to cook the other side for the same time, or until the turkey is cooked through. Set aside to rest.

2 Make the tabbouleh by mixing the bulgur wheat, parsley, mint, and dill in a bowl, then season with salt and pepper to taste. Stir in the pomegranate seeds, sumac, and lemon juice.

3 Slice the turkey diagonally into strips, then transfer the turkey and the tabbouleh to a serving bowl. Add the spinach, then scatter over the pistachios and harissa.

the BUILD

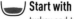 **Start with** turkey and tabbouleh

 Add in pistachios and harissa

 Finish with spinach leaves

DF **GF** **VG**

UNDER 600 CALS

Green lentils & brown rice
with tomato & chili salsa

prep **10 MIN**   cook **15 MIN**

A tangy, fruity salsa works beautifully in this bowl of earthy lentils, hearty rice, and crunchy roasted broccoli.

Calories **438**	Cholesterol **0mg**	Dietary fiber **11.5g**
Total fat **6g**	Sodium **18mg**	Sugars **18.5g**
Saturated fat **1g**	Carbohydrates **74g**	Protein **16.5g**

the INGREDIENTS

½ cup brown rice

sea salt and freshly ground black pepper

1 cup broccoli florets

1 tsp olive oil

½ cup cooked green lentils

1 tsp raisins

handful of dill, finely chopped

1 orange, half juiced, half peeled and segmented

a few cilantro leaves

For the salsa

2 tomatoes, seeds removed, and flesh chopped

½ red onion, finely chopped

½ red chili pepper, finely chopped

small handful of cilantro leaves

juice of ½ lime

1 tsp olive oil

the PREP

1 Put the rice and a pinch of sea salt in a saucepan with 1½ cups of water. Bring to a boil, then reduce the heat to a gentle simmer, cover, and cook for 10–15 minutes, or according to the package instructions, until the water is absorbed and the rice tender. Set aside, keeping the lid on.

2 Meanwhile, preheat the oven to 400°F (200°C). Mix the broccoli and olive oil in a roasting pan, seasoning with salt and pepper. Roast for 10–15 minutes, or until the broccoli begins to turn golden brown. Set aside.

3 Make the salsa by mixing the tomatoes, red onion, red chili pepper, cilantro leaves, lime juice, and olive oil in a bowl, seasoning with salt and pepper. (This makes 2 portions. Store the extra portion in an airtight container in the fridge for up to 3 days.)

4 Mix the green lentils, raisins, dill, and orange juice in a bowl, and season with salt and pepper.

5 Transfer the rice to a serving bowl, then add the lentil mixture and broccoli. Spoon in the salsa, scatter with the orange segments, and sprinkle with the cilantro leaves.

the BUILD

 Start with
brown rice, lentil mixture, and broccoli

 Add in
tomato-chili pepper salsa

 Finish with
orange segments and cilantro leaves

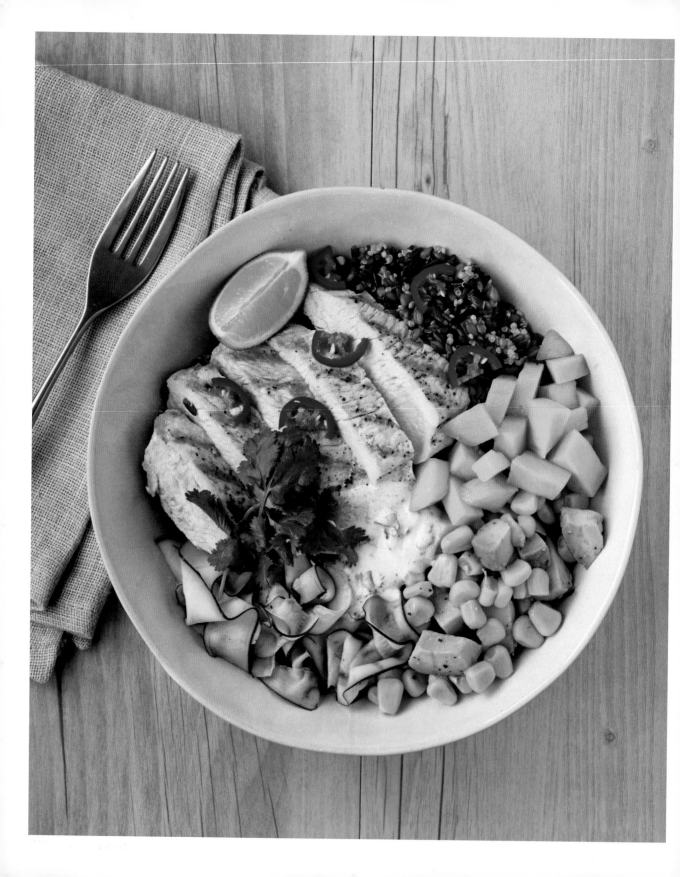

UNDER
600
CALS

Turkey & mango
with corn & avocado salsa

prep **15 MIN**   cook **10 MIN**

Lean turkey works well with the sweet, juicy mango and grilled zucchini ribbons in this bowl.

Calories **583**	Cholesterol **3.4mg**	Dietary fiber **14g**
Total fat **28g**	Sodium **43mg**	Sugars **15g**
Saturated fat **4.5g**	Carbohydrates **44g**	Protein **32g**

the INGREDIENTS

4½ oz (125g) turkey breast

1 tsp olive oil

sea salt and freshly ground black pepper

1 cup zucchini, peeled into ribbons with a vegetable peeler

½ avocado

juice of 1 lemon

⅓ cup sweet corn

¾ cup cooked spelt, quinoa, red rice, and wild rice mix, or other cooked grain mix

⅓ cup mango, chopped

a few cilantro leaves

¼ red chili pepper, sliced (optional)

lime wedge (optional)

For the dressing

1 tsp extra virgin olive oil

¼ tsp white wine vinegar

2 tsp 0% fat plain Greek yogurt

handful of cilantro leaves, finely chopped

the PREP

1 Coat the turkey breast with ½ tsp of the olive oil, and rub with salt and pepper.

2 Heat a griddle pan on high heat, then toss the zucchini with the remaining ½ tsp of olive oil and some salt and pepper. Put the zucchini in the pan, cook for 1 minute on each side, then remove from the pan and set aside. Clean and reheat the griddle pan, then add the turkey to the hot pan and cook for 3–4 minutes on each side or until cooked through. Allow to rest for 5 minutes.

3 Make the dressing by mixing the extra virgin olive oil, white wine vinegar, Greek yogurt, and cilantro leaves in a bowl, then season with salt and pepper.

4 Chop the avocado and toss in another bowl with the lemon juice to prevent discoloration, then add the sweet corn and season with salt and pepper.

5 Slice the turkey into strips and place in a serving bowl, then add the zucchini, sweet corn mixture, spelt mix, and mango. Spoon on the dressing, sprinkle over the cilantro leaves and red chili pepper (if using), and add the lime wedge (if using), to squeeze over.

the BUILD

 Start with
turkey, zucchini, sweet corn mixture, spelt mix, and mango

 Add in
yogurt dressing, cilantro leaves, and red chili pepper

 Finish with
lime wedge

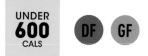

UNDER 600 CALS · **DF** · **GF**

Turkey & whole grains
with pineapple & coconut

prep **10 MIN**   cook **15 MIN**

Sweet and savory mixes never fail to satisfy, while hot harissa perks up everything in this soothing bowl.

Calories **429**	Cholesterol **34g**	Dietary fiber **8.5g**
Total fat **16g**	Sodium **426mg**	Sugars **7.5g**
Saturated fat **7.5g**	Carbohydrates **43g**	Protein **23.5g**

the INGREDIENTS

4½ oz (125g) turkey breast

sea salt and black peppercorns

1 cup cooked quinoa and brown rice mix

½ cup pineapple, finely chopped

a few thyme leaves

½ tsp harissa

small handful of mint leaves, half chopped, the rest left whole

½ cup fresh coconut chunks

pinch of chia seeds

1 green onion, white part only, finely shredded, soaked in cold water for 10 minutes (optional)

the PREP

1   Put the turkey breast in a saucepan, cover with cold water, season with sea salt, and add a few black peppercorns. Bring to a boil, then reduce the heat to a simmer and cook for 15 minutes or until the turkey is cooked through and the juices run clear when it is pierced with a sharp knife. Remove the turkey from the saucepan using a slotted spoon and set aside. Once it has cooled, shred it.

2   Combine the quinoa and brown rice mix, pineapple, thyme leaves, ¼ tsp of the harissa, and the chopped mint leaves in a bowl.

3   Put the turkey in a serving bowl, then add the quinoa and brown rice mixture, the coconut, and remaining ¼ tsp of harissa. Sprinkle over the chia seeds, the whole mint leaves, and the green onion.

the BUILD

 Start with
turkey

 Add in
quinoa and brown rice mixture, coconut, and harissa

 Finish with
chia seeds, mint leaves, and green onion

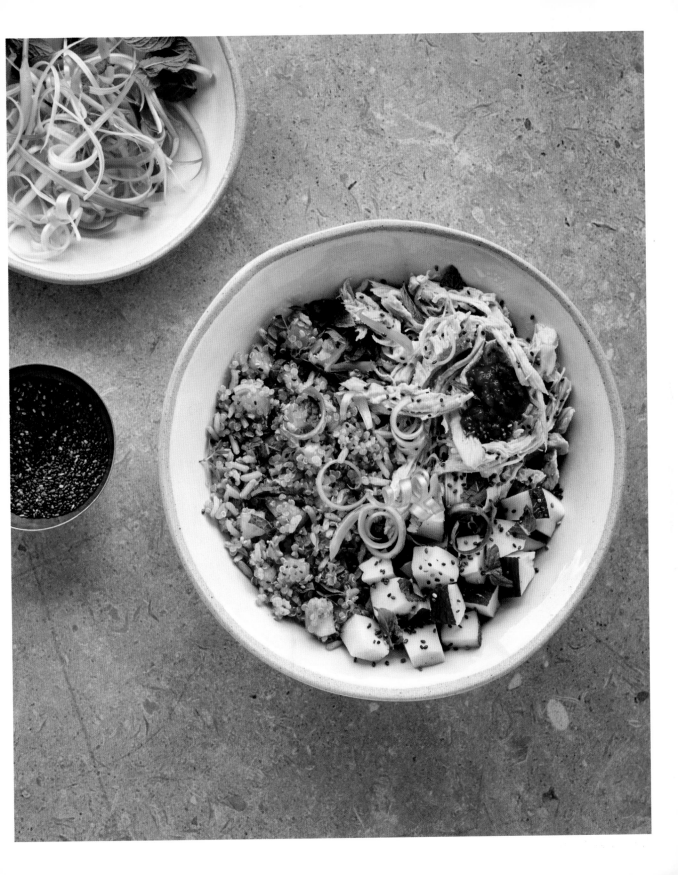

UNDER
600
CALS

Roasted cauliflower couscous
with raisin salsa & tahini

prep **15 MIN**   cook **15 MIN**

Roasting cauliflower gives it a nutty sweetness; when chopped, it makes a low-carb alternative to couscous.

Calories **427**	Cholesterol **0mg**	Dietary fiber **16g**
Total fat **16g**	Sodium **38mg**	Sugars **23g**
Saturated fat **2.5g**	Carbohydrates **42g**	Protein **22g**

the INGREDIENTS

1 cup cauliflower florets

1 tsp olive oil

sea salt and freshly ground black pepper

1 tsp sumac

½ cup cooked chickpeas

1 tsp pumpkin seeds

handful of mint leaves

1 tsp chopped pistachios

¼ green chili pepper, finely sliced

lemon wedge (optional)

For the salsa

3 tbsp raisins

1 tsp baby capers

1 tomato, finely chopped

½ green onion, white part only, finely chopped

For the dressing

1 tbsp 0% fat plain Greek yogurt

2 tsp tahini

juice of ¼ lemon

the PREP

1 Preheat the oven to 400°F (200°C). Mix the cauliflower and olive oil in a roasting pan, seasoning with salt and pepper. Roast for 10–15 minutes or until the cauliflower starts to turn golden brown and is tender. Let it cool for 2–3 minutes, then chop it coarsely in a food processor with the sumac until it becomes the texture of couscous. Set aside.

2 Make the salsa by mixing the raisins, baby capers, tomato, and green onion in a bowl, seasoning with salt and pepper. Set aside.

3 Make the dressing by mixing the Greek yogurt, tahini, and lemon juice in a bowl, seasoning with salt to taste. (This makes 2 servings. Store the extra serving in an airtight container in the fridge for up to 2 days.)

4 Spoon the cauliflower into a serving bowl, then add the chickpeas, raisin salsa, and tahini dressing. Sprinkle with the pumpkin seeds, mint leaves, pistachios, and green chili pepper, and add the lemon wedge (if using) to squeeze over.

the BUILD

 Start with
cauliflower, chickpeas, raisin salsa, and tahini dressing

 Add in
pumpkin seeds, mint leaves, pistachios, and green chili pepper

Finish with
lemon wedge

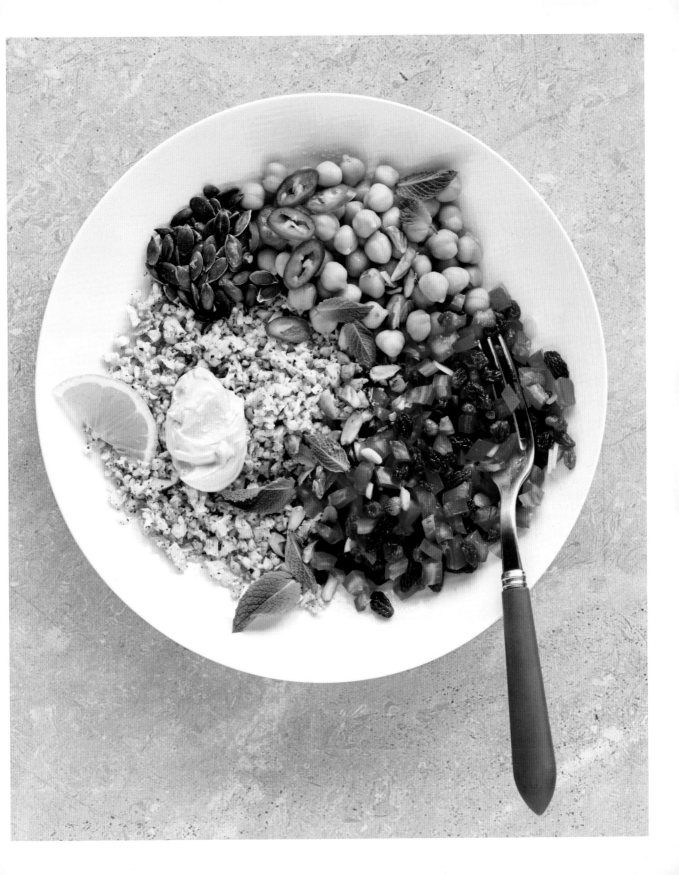

DF GF VG

Green lentils & sour cherries
with cucumber & zucchini

prep **5 MIN**   cook **10 MIN**

Lentils and lima beans offer optimum nutrients here, with cucumber for crunch, and cherry and mint for zing.

Calories **317**	Cholesterol **0mg**	Dietary fiber **15g**
Total fat **8.5g**	Sodium **19mg**	Sugars **9g**
Saturated fat **1g**	Carbohydrates **35g**	Protein **17.5g**

the INGREDIENTS

1 cup fine green beans, trimmed

sea salt and freshly ground black pepper

1 tsp olive oil

1 zucchini, halved lengthways, and cut into small batons

handful of dill, finely chopped

½ cup cooked lima beans

handful of mint leaves, chopped, plus a few whole leaves to serve

½ cup cooked green lentils

1 tsp dried sour cherries, chopped

½ cucumber, halved lengthwise, and sliced

½ tsp white wine vinegar

For the dressing

1 tsp extra virgin olive oil

1 tsp white wine vinegar

pinch of paprika

the PREP

1 Put the green beans in a saucepan of boiling salted water and cook for about 4 minutes, then drain, refresh with cold water, drain again, and set aside.

2 Heat the olive oil in a frying pan on medium heat, then add the zucchini and some salt and pepper. Cook for 4 minutes, stirring regularly, then add the green beans and dill, cooking for 2 more minutes. Set aside.

3 Make the dressing by mixing the extra virgin olive oil, white wine vinegar, and paprika in a bowl, then seasoning with salt and pepper to taste. Stir in the lima beans and chopped mint.

4 Mix the green lentils and dried sour cherries in another bowl, and season with salt and pepper.

5 Combine the cucumber, white wine vinegar, and mint leaves in a bowl, again seasoning with salt and pepper.

6 Spoon the green lentils and cherries mixture into a serving bowl, then add the zucchini and green bean mixture and the lima bean mixture, and spoon on the cucumber and mint mixture.

the BUILD

 Start with
green lentils and cherries mixture

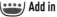 **Add in**
zucchini and green bean mixture and lima beans

 Finish with
cucumber and mint mixture

DF **VG** **UNDER 400 CALS**

Ginger & soy brown rice
with crispy stir-fried tofu

prep **5 MIN**   cook **5 MIN**

Tofu becomes crispy when cooked in olive oil, allowing it to soak up all the delicious Asian flavors in this bowl.

Calories **398**	Cholesterol **0mg**	Dietary fiber **6.5g**
Total fat **14.5g**	Sodium **575mg**	Sugars **7.5g**
Saturated fat **2.5g**	Carbohydrates **43g**	Protein **21g**

the INGREDIENTS

1 tsp olive oil

1 cup firm tofu, cut into small cubes

1 tsp dark soy sauce

1 cup cooked brown rice

¼ green onion, finely chopped

1-in (2.5cm) piece of fresh ginger, peeled and grated

3 radishes, trimmed and sliced

½ cup sugar snap peas, finely sliced diagonally

pinch of sesame seeds

a few cilantro leaves

For the dressing

1 tsp dark soy sauce

juice of ½ lemon

½ tsp mirin rice wine

sea salt and freshly ground black pepper

the PREP

1 Heat the olive oil in a wok or a frying pan on medium heat. Mix the tofu and dark soy sauce in a bowl, then add to the hot wok or pan. Cook for 3–5 minutes, stirring often, or until the tofu is golden brown and crispy. Remove with a slotted spoon, and place it on a plate lined with a paper towel to absorb excess olive oil.

2 Make the dressing by mixing the dark soy sauce, lemon juice, and mirin in a bowl, seasoning with salt and pepper.

3 Mix the brown rice, green onion, ginger, and half the dressing in a bowl. Spoon the rice mixture into a serving bowl, then add the tofu, radishes, and sugar snap peas. Scatter over the sesame seeds and cilantro leaves, then drizzle with the remaining dressing.

the BUILD

 Start with
brown rice, tofu, radishes, and sugar snap peas

 Add in
sesame seeds and cilantro leaves

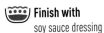 **Finish with**
soy sauce dressing

Spelt, kale & broccoli
with lima beans & peas

prep **5 MIN**   cook **10 MIN**

Spelt is a heritage wheat grain that teams well with green vegetables for a nutritious meal.

Calories **529**	Cholesterol **0mg**	Dietary fiber **18g**
Total fat **20g**	Sodium **190mg**	Sugars **11g**
Saturated fat **3.5g**	Carbohydrates **55g**	Protein **24g**

the INGREDIENTS

1 cup broccoli florets

1 tsp olive oil

1 tsp ground turmeric

sea salt and freshly ground black pepper

1½ cups kale, coarse stalks removed, leaves chopped

1 cup peas, defrosted if frozen

½ cup cooked lima beans

½ cup cooked spelt

1 tomato, halved, seeds removed, and flesh chopped

2 tsp 0% fat plain Greek yogurt

6 cashews, roughly chopped

½ green chili pepper, finely chopped

pinch of nigella seeds

lime wedge (optional)

the PREP

1   Preheat the oven to 400°F (200°C) and mix the broccoli, olive oil, and turmeric in a roasting pan, seasoning with salt and pepper. Roast for 10 minutes or until the broccoli starts to turn golden brown.

2   Meanwhile, steam the kale over boiling water for 10 minutes, then mix with the peas, lima beans, and broccoli.

3   Spoon the spelt into a serving bowl, then add the broccoli mixture, tomato, and Greek yogurt. Sprinkle with the cashews, green chili pepper, and nigella seeds, and add the lime wedge (if using), to squeeze over the bowl.

the BUILD

 Start with
spelt

 Add in
broccoli and lima bean mixture, tomato, and Greek yogurt

 Finish with
cashews, green chili pepper, nigella seeds, and lime wedge

DF VG

UNDER **400** CALS

Spelt & roasted cauliflower
with sumac dressing

prep **15 MIN**   cook **15 MIN**

Middle Eastern ingredients mingle here with earthy lentils for protein and healthy green spinach for iron.

Calories **360**	Cholesterol **0mg**	Dietary fiber **9g**
Total fat **14g**	Sodium **149mg**	Sugars **14g**
Saturated fat **2g**	Carbohydrates **41g**	Protein **13g**

the INGREDIENTS

1 tsp barberries

½ small cauliflower, broken into florets

1 tsp olive oil

sea salt and freshly ground black pepper

2 cups spinach leaves

½ red onion, finely sliced

1 tsp capers

½ cup cooked spelt

1 tsp flaked almonds, toasted (see p129)

1 tsp pomegranate seeds

handful of dill leaves, finely chopped

For the dressing

1 tsp extra virgin olive oil

1 tsp white wine vinegar

pinch of sumac

the PREP

1 Preheat the oven to 400°F (200°C). Put the barberries in a cup, cover with water, and soak for 5 minutes, then drain.

2 Mix the cauliflower and olive oil in a roasting pan, seasoning with salt and pepper. Roast for 10–15 minutes or until the cauliflower turns golden brown. Remove the pan from the oven, add the cauliflower to a bowl, and leave to cool for 2–3 minutes, then add the spinach, red onion, and capers.

3 Make the dressing by whisking the extra virgin olive oil, white wine vinegar, and sumac in a bowl, seasoning with salt and pepper.

4 Spoon the spelt into a serving bowl, then add the cauliflower mixture. Scatter over the almonds, barberries, pomegranate seeds, and dill leaves, and drizzle with the sumac dressing.

the BUILD

 Start with
spelt and
cauliflower mixture

 Add in
almonds, barberries,
pomegranate seeds,
and dill leaves

 Finish with
sumac dressing

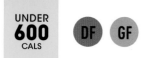

UNDER 600 CALS **DF** **GF**

Seared tuna
with ginger dressing & citrus

prep **10 MIN**   cook **5 MIN**

Citrus fruits add a tang without piling on calories, and work especially well with rice and tuna.

Calories **587**	Cholesterol **35mg**	Dietary fiber **11g**
Total fat **21g**	Sodium **80mg**	Sugars **20g**
Saturated fat **4g**	Carbohydrates **57g**	Protein **37g**

the INGREDIENTS

3½ oz (100g) tuna steak

1 tsp olive oil

sea salt and freshly ground black pepper

1 pink grapefruit, peeled

1 orange, peeled

½ small avocado

1 cup cooked brown rice

½ cup frozen edamame, defrosted

handful of cress

For the dressing

1 tsp extra virgin olive oil

½ tsp white wine vinegar

½-in (1.5cm) piece of fresh ginger, peeled and grated or finely chopped

the PREP

1 Brush the tuna steak with olive oil and season with salt and pepper. Heat a griddle pan on high, put the tuna on it, and cook undisturbed for 1–2 minutes on each side. (The middle should stay pink.) Remove it from the pan and let it rest for 5 minutes, then cut into bite-sized chunks.

2 Make the dressing by mixing the extra virgin olive oil, white wine vinegar, and ginger in a bowl, seasoning with salt and pepper to taste.

3 Segment the grapefruit and orange over a bowl, to collect excess juice. Roughly chop the avocado, then toss it in the citrus juice, to prevent discoloration.

4 Put the brown rice in a serving bowl, then add the tuna, avocado, edamame, and cress. Scatter over the grapefruit and orange segments and drizzle with the ginger dressing.

the BUILD

 Start with
brown rice

 Add in
tuna, avocado,
edamame,
and cress

 Finish with
grapefruit segments,
orange segments,
and ginger dressing

DF **GF** UNDER **600** CALS

Grilled squid & fennel
with tomato guacamole

prep **15 MIN**   cook **15 MIN**

Grilled squid is a great low-calorie food, delicious paired with fennel and tomato guacamole.

Calories **461**	Cholesterol **225mg**	Dietary fiber **8g**
Total fat **21g**	Sodium **136mg**	Sugars **3g**
Saturated fat **4.5g**	Carbohydrates **41g**	Protein **23g**

the INGREDIENTS

¼ fennel bulb, sliced lengthwise

1 tsp olive oil

handful of flat-leaf parsley, finely chopped

3½oz (100g) baby squid, bodies opened and scored into a crisscross on the insides

pinch of red pepper flakes

1 cup cooked brown rice

handful of arugula

For the guacamole

1 avocado

1 tomato, finely chopped

juice from 1 lime

handful of cilantro leaves, finely chopped, plus whole leaves to serve

sea salt and freshly ground black pepper

the PREP

1   Make the guacamole. Peel, pit, and coarsely mash the avocado with the tomato, lime juice, and chopped cilantro leaves in a bowl, seasoning with salt and pepper. (This makes 2 portions. Store the extra portion in an airtight container in the fridge for up to 2 days.)

2   Toss the fennel in ½ tsp of the olive oil in a bowl, and season with salt and pepper. Heat a griddle pan on high heat, place the fennel in the pan, and cook for 5 minutes on each side, or until charred lines appear. Remove the fennel from the pan, return it to the bowl, stir in the flat-leaf parsley, and set aside. Wipe the griddle pan clean.

3   Mix the squid with the remaining ½ tsp of olive oil in a bowl, add the red pepper flakes, and season with salt and pepper. Heat the cleaned griddle pan on high heat. Put in the squid, cook for 2 minutes on each side or until it begins to char, then remove.

4   Spoon the brown rice into a serving bowl, then add the arugula, fennel, and squid. Spoon on the guacamole and sprinkle with the whole cilantro leaves.

the BUILD

 Start with
brown rice

 Add in
arugula, fennel, and squid

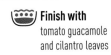 **Finish with**
tomato guacamole and cilantro leaves

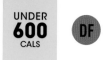

Chicken & egg oyakodon
with jasmine rice

prep **15 MIN**   cook **15 MIN**

This super-healthy comfort food mixes rice and tender chicken in a nourishing broth with a seaweed booster.

Calories **437**	Cholesterol **301mg**	Dietary fiber **5g**
Total fat **7g**	Sodium **804mg**	Sugars **6g**
Saturated fat **2g**	Carbohydrates **55g**	Protein **45g**

the INGREDIENTS

2 green onions, trimmed, green parts only, 1 shredded lengthwise, 1 finely sliced

½ cup jasmine rice

sea salt

4½ oz (125g) skinless chicken breast

¼ red onion, sliced

1 piece of dried wakame (optional)

2 tsp dark soy sauce

1 egg, lightly beaten

½ sheet nori, cut into fine strips

handful of cilantro leaves

the PREP

1 Soak the shredded green onion in ice-cold water for 10 minutes, or longer if possible, then drain and pat dry.

2 Put the jasmine rice and some sea salt in a saucepan with ½ cup of water. Bring to a boil, then reduce the heat to a gentle simmer, cover, and cook for 15 minutes, or until the water has been absorbed and the rice is tender. Set aside, keeping the lid on.

3 Meanwhile, put the chicken in a saucepan, cover with water, and season with some sea salt, then add the red onion, wakame (if using), and dark soy sauce. Bring to a boil, then reduce the heat to a gentle simmer, cover, and cook for 5–10 minutes, or until the chicken is cooked and the juices run clear when it is pierced with a sharp knife.

4 Remove the chicken from the pan, cut it into chunks, and put them in a frying pan, along with a few ladles of the poaching liquid, and the finely sliced green onion. Bring to a gentle simmer, then pour the beaten egg over it, cover, and cook for 2 minutes, or until the egg starts to set.

5 Spoon the rice into a serving bowl, then add the chicken and egg mixture (including the poaching liquid), and the nori. Scatter with the shredded green onion, and the cilantro leaves.

the BUILD

 Start with
jasmine rice

 Add in
chicken and egg mixture

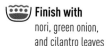 **Finish with**
nori, green onion, and cilantro leaves

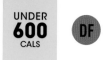
UNDER
600
CALS

DF

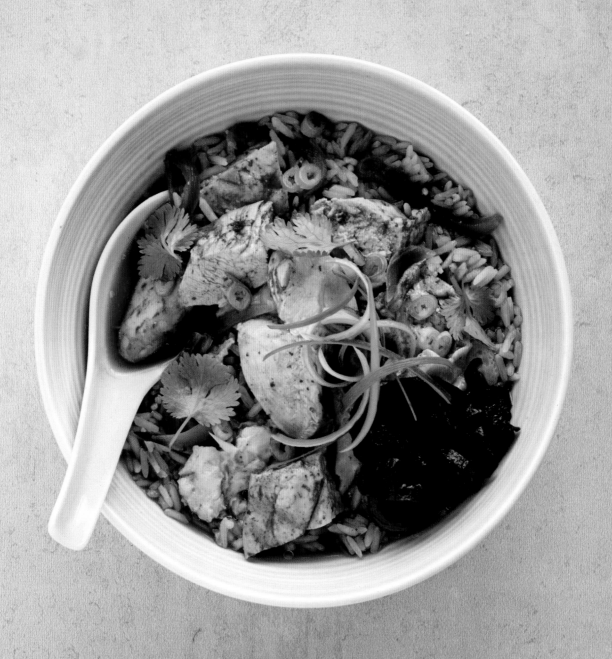

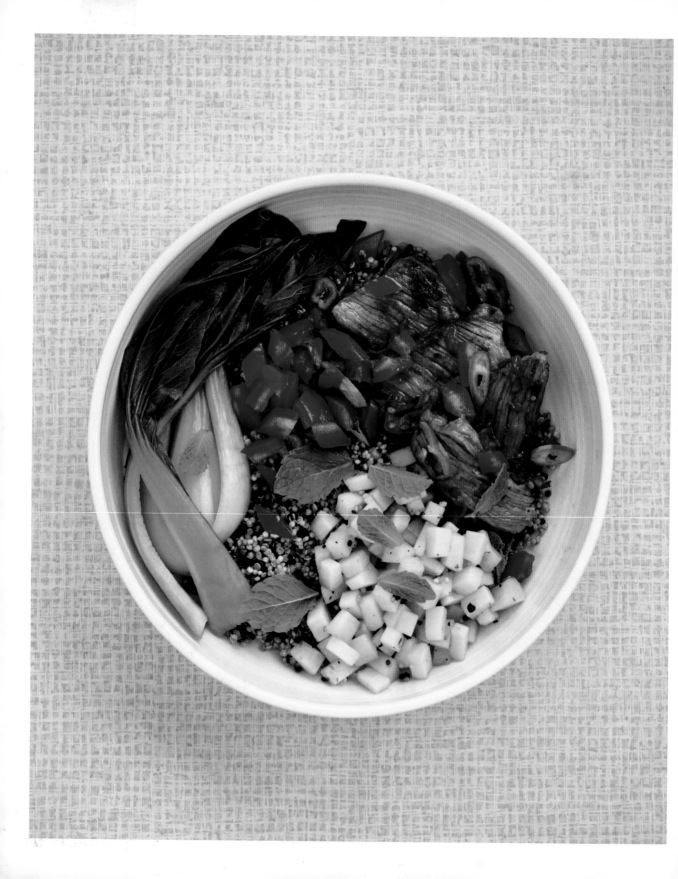

Hot & sour pork
with steamed bok choi

prep **15 MIN** cook **15 MIN**

A sweet marinade adds great flavors to the pork and creates a wonderfully tender and delicious bowl.

Calories **298**	Cholesterol **79mg**	Dietary fiber **6g**
Total fat **7g**	Sodium **150mg**	Sugars **8g**
Saturated fat **2g**	Carbohydrates **23g**	Protein **34g**

the INGREDIENTS

4½ oz (125g) pork tenderloin, sliced into 4–5 thin slices

⅓ cup white, black, and red quinoa mix

¼ cup cucumber, peeled, seeds removed, and finely chopped

1 tsp rice vinegar

¼ tsp peeled and grated fresh ginger

1 cup bok choi

½ tomato, seeds removed, and flesh finely chopped

¼ green chili pepper, finely sliced

a few fresh mint leaves (optional)

lime wedges (optional)

For the marinade

1 tsp mirin rice vinegar

2 tsp rice vinegar

¼ tsp honey

½ tomato, finely chopped

1 garlic clove, grated

¼ red chili pepper, finely chopped

sea salt and freshly ground black pepper

the PREP

1 Make the marinade by mixing the mirin, rice vinegar, honey, tomato, garlic, red chili pepper, and salt and pepper to taste in a bowl. Add the pork, and allow it to marinate for 10 minutes.

2 Put the quinoa mix and some sea salt in a saucepan with ⅔ cup of water. Bring to a boil, then cover and cook for 10 minutes, or until the water is absorbed and the quinoa is tender. Set aside, keeping the lid on.

3 Meanwhile, toss the cucumber, rice vinegar, and ginger in a bowl, seasoning with salt and pepper.

4 Heat a griddle pan on high heat, then add the pork and marinade. Cook for 3 minutes on each side, or until golden brown, then set aside.

5 At the same time, steam the bok choi for 4 minutes.

6 Spoon the quinoa mix into a serving bowl, then add the pork and bok choi. Next, add the cucumber mixture, tomato, and green chilim pepper. Scatter with the mint leaves and add the lime wedges (if using), to squeeze over.

the BUILD

 Start with
quinoa mix

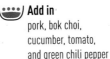 **Add in**
pork, bok choi, cucumber, tomato, and green chili pepper

 Finish with
mint leaves and lime wedges

UNDER **300** CALS

 DF GF VG

Zucchini & carrot spaghetti
with cherry tomato sauce

prep **15 MIN**   cook **10 MIN**

Eliminate heavy carbs with this healthy take on spaghetti. A spiralizer makes cutting the vegetables much easier.

Calories **116**	Cholesterol **0mg**	Dietary fiber **6g**
Total fat **4.5g**	Sodium **36mg**	Sugars **10g**
Saturated fat **0.8g**	Carbohydrates **11g**	Protein **5g**

the INGREDIENTS

1 tsp olive oil

¼ cup zucchini, sliced, spiralized, or cut into fine strips

sea salt and freshly ground black pepper

pinch of red pepper flakes

pinch of dried oregano

1 garlic clove, finely chopped

½ cup carrot, sliced, and spiralized, or cut into fine strips

For the sauce

8 cherry tomatoes, halved

1 tsp olive oil

pinch of sumac

handful of basil leaves, half roughly chopped, the rest left whole

the PREP

1 Heat the olive oil in a nonstick frying pan on medium heat, put the zucchini in the pan, and season with some salt and pepper. Toss the zucchini around the pan for a few seconds, then add the red pepper flakes, oregano, and garlic, and cook for 2–3 minutes.

2 Add the carrot to the pan, tossing to coat, and cook for 2 more minutes or until both vegetables are tender but still retain some bite.

3 Meanwhile, make the sauce by tossing the cherry tomatoes in olive oil, sumac, and salt and pepper to taste in a bowl. Place a frying pan on high heat and, when it's hot, add the tomato mixture and cook for 4–5 minutes, squashing the tomatoes a little with a wooden spoon. (Add a tiny amount of hot water if there's not much juice.) Stir in the chopped basil leaves.

4 Transfer the vegetable spaghetti to a serving bowl, then spoon on the cherry tomato sauce and scatter over the whole basil leaves.

the BUILD

 Start with zucchini and carrot spaghetti

 Add in cherry tomato sauce

 Finish with basil leaves

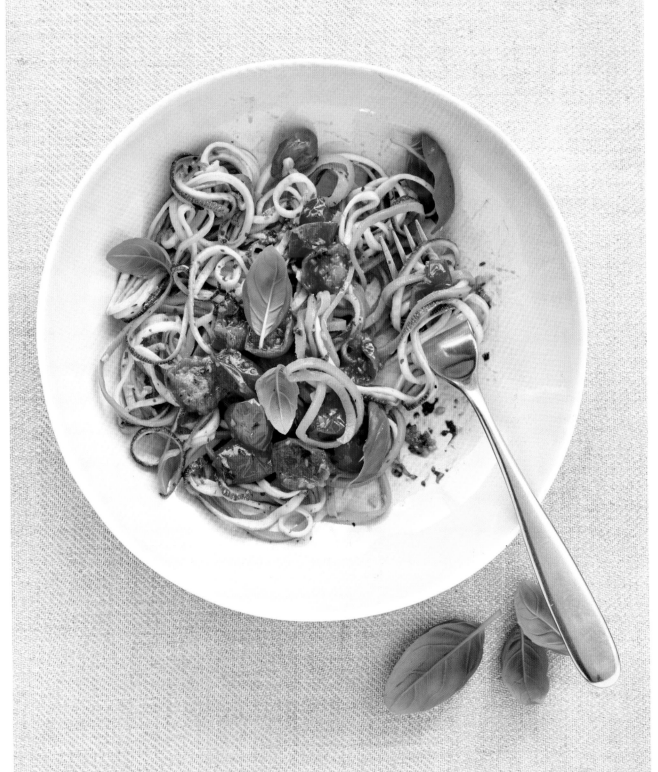

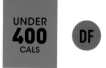

UNDER 400 CALS · DF

Salmon & bok choi
with ginger rice & pineapple

prep 15 MIN   cook 15 MIN

Red chili pepper, pineapple, and salmon chunks in lime and soy sauce fuse together some great tastes.

Calories **350**	Cholesterol **85mg**	Dietary fiber **7g**
Total fat **19g**	Sodium **403mg**	Sugars **7.5g**
Saturated fat **3.5g**	Carbohydrates **11g**	Protein **30g**

the INGREDIENTS

4½ oz (125g) salmon fillet, skinned

2 heads of bok choi, sliced lengthwise

1 cup green beans

8 almonds, roughly chopped

½ cup cooked brown rice

½-in (1.5cm) piece of fresh ginger, peeled and grated

⅓ cup fresh pineapple, diced

¼ red chili pepper, finely chopped

1 green onion, green part only, finely sliced

a few cilantro leaves (optional)

For the marinade

juice of ½ lime

1 tsp dark soy sauce

1 tsp mirin rice wine

½-in (1.5cm) piece of lemongrass, outer layer trimmed, inner part finely sliced

sea salt and freshly ground black pepper

the PREP

1 Make the marinade by whisking the lime juice, dark soy sauce, mirin, and lemongrass in a bowl, seasoning with salt and pepper. Put the salmon in a shallow bowl, coat it with the marinade, and leave to marinate for 10 minutes.

2 Heat a nonstick griddle pan on high heat, add the salmon, and drizzle the marinade on top. Cook for 3–4 minutes on each side, or until cooked through. Leave to rest for 5 minutes, then cut into chunks.

3 Meanwhile, steam the bok choi over boiling water for 5–6 minutes, or until tender. Set aside.

4 Put the green beans in a saucepan of boiling salted water. Cook for 4 minutes or until tender. Drain, refresh with cold water, and drain again. Toss with the almonds.

5 Mix the brown rice and ginger, season with salt and pepper, then spoon into a serving bowl. Add the bok choi, green beans, salmon, and pineapple, then sprinkle with the red chili pepper, green onion, and cilantro leaves (if using).

the BUILD

 Start with
brown rice and ginger

 Add in
bok choi, green beans, salmon, and pineapple

 Finish with
red chili pepper, green onion, and cilantro leaves

DF VG

UNDER **600** CALS

Eggplant & tofu
with green bean relish

prep **10 MIN**   cook **10 MIN**

The tofu and eggplant in this bowl harmonize to absorb all the flavors of the simple soy sauce–based dressing.

Calories **504**	Cholesterol **0mg**	Dietary fiber **11g**
Total fat **13g**	Sodium **616mg**	Sugars **42g**
Saturated fat **2g**	Carbohydrates **70g**	Protein **21g**

the INGREDIENTS

¼ eggplant, cut into cubes

½ cup firm tofu, cut into cubes

1 tsp dark soy sauce

1 tsp mirin rice wine

juice of ½ lime

pinch of red pepper flakes

sea salt and freshly ground black pepper

½ cup cooked green lentils

⅓ cup cooked red and white quinoa

handful of flat-leaf parsley, chopped

3 dates, finely chopped

1 cup spinach leaves

1 tsp pumpkin seeds

a few mint leaves

For the dressing

1 tsp extra virgin olive oil

1 tsp white wine vinegar

1 tsp dark soy sauce

juice of ½ orange

For the relish

1 cup green beans

¼ red onion, finely chopped

3 cherry tomatoes, finely chopped

the PREP

1 Put the eggplant and tofu in a bowl, then stir in the dark soy sauce, mirin, lime juice, and red pepper flakes. Season to taste with salt and pepper, then leave to marinate.

2 Mix the green lentils, quinoa, flat-leaf parsley, and dates in a bowl, then season with salt and pepper. Set aside.

3 Make the dressing by whisking the extra virgin olive oil, white wine vinegar, dark soy sauce, and orange juice in another bowl, seasoning with salt and pepper. Set aside.

4 Make the relish: cook the green beans in a saucepan of boiling salted water for 5 minutes, drain, then chop. Mix with the red onion, cherry tomatoes, and some salt and pepper in a bowl. (This makes 2 portions. Store the extra portion in an airtight container in the fridge for up to 3 days.)

5 Heat a griddle pan on medium heat; add the eggplant, tofu, and marinade; and cook undisturbed for 2–3 minutes on each side, or until golden brown.

6 Transfer the green lentil mixture into a serving bowl, then add the eggplant, tofu, and spinach. Spoon in the green bean relish, and drizzle with the dressing. Add the pumpkin seeds on top, along with the mint leaves.

the BUILD

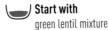

Start with
green lentil mixture

Add in
eggplant, tofu, spinach leaves, and green bean relish

Finish with
orange juice dressing, pumpkin seeds, and mint leaves

Relaxed
meals

These recipes might take a little more time and effort to prep and cook, but as you enjoy that first bite, you'd never guess you're eating a meal designed to help you lose weight.

UNDER 600 CALS **DF** **GF**

Pickled herring & cranberries
with horseradish dressing

prep **10 MIN**   cook **30 MIN**

A nutty rice salad rounds off the piquant ingredients in this bowl, with its strong, hot dressing.

Calories **571**	Cholesterol **18mg**	Dietary fiber **6g**
Total fat **12.5g**	Sodium **400mg**	Sugars **17g**
Saturated fat **1.5g**	Carbohydrates **91g**	Protein **21g**

the INGREDIENTS

½ cup red rice and wild rice mix

sea salt and freshly ground black pepper

½ Gala apple

juice of 1 lemon

⅓ cup pickled herring

4 radishes, finely sliced

small handful of watercress

2 tsp dried cranberries

pinch of poppy seeds

For the dressing

2 tsp extra virgin olive oil

1 tsp hot horseradish sauce,
   or freshly grated horseradish

juice of ¼ lemon

the PREP

1 Put the rice and some sea salt in a saucepan with 1½ cups of water, and cook for 20–30 minutes or until tender. Drain and set aside.

2 Make the dressing by mixing the extra virgin olive oil, hot horseradish sauce, and lemon juice from ¼ lemon in a bowl, and season with salt and pepper to taste.

3 Core and slice the apple, then toss in the lemon juice from 1 lemon to prevent discoloration.

4 Put the rice and the pickled herring in a serving bowl, then add the apple, radishes, and watercress. Sprinkle the cranberries and poppy seeds on the apple and radishes, and drizzle in the dressing.

the BUILD

 Start with
rice mix and
pickled herring

 Add in
apple, radishes,
and watercress

 Finish with
cranberries,
poppy seeds, and
horseradish dressing

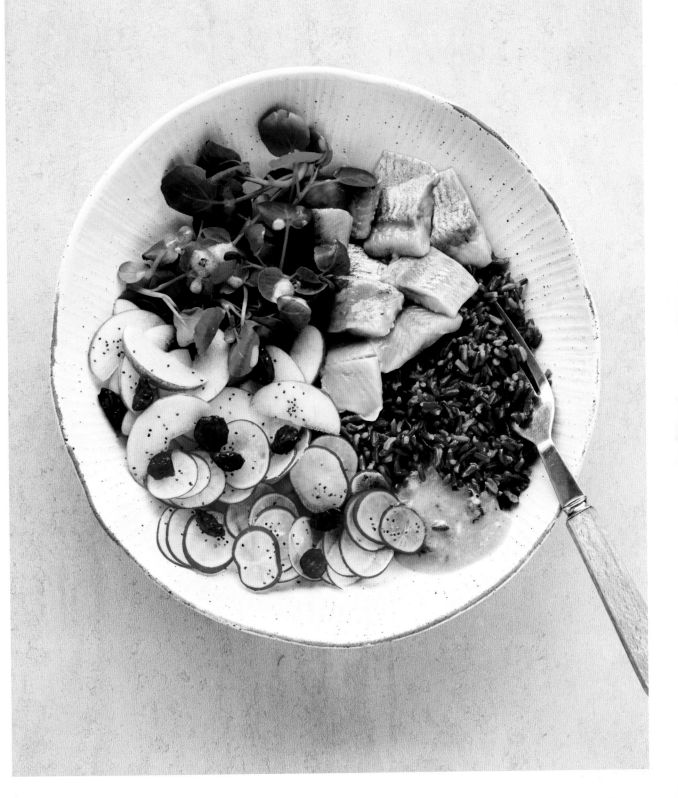

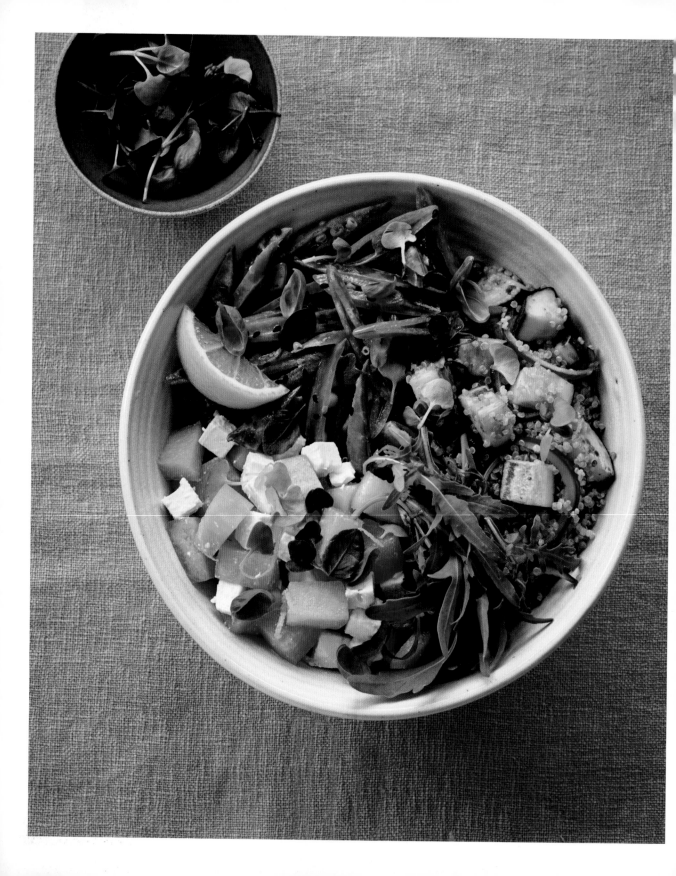

GF UNDER **400** CALS

Quinoa, melon, & feta
with mustard dressing

prep **15 MIN**   cook **25 MIN**

This is a power bowl packed with sweet melon, salty feta, nutty quinoa, and tangy mustard dressing.

Calories **384**	Cholesterol **28mg**	Dietary fiber **8g**
Total fat **17g**	Sodium **479mg**	Sugars **13g**
Saturated fat **7g**	Carbohydrates **36g**	Protein **19g**

the INGREDIENTS

1 cup quinoa

sea salt and freshly ground black pepper

1 tsp olive oil

1 cup zucchini, finely chopped

¼ red onion, finely chopped

finely grated zest of 1 lemon

½ garlic clove, finely chopped

pinch of paprika

⅓ cup feta cheese, cubed

⅓ cup cantaloupe, cubed

1 cup sugar snap peas, sliced diagonally

pinch of black sesame seeds

handful of arugula

a few green and/or purple basil leaves (optional)

lemon wedge (optional)

For the dressing

1 tsp extra virgin olive oil

1 tsp apple cider vinegar

½ tsp Dijon mustard

the PREP

1 Put the quinoa and some sea salt in a saucepan with 2¼ cups of water. Bring to a boil, then reduce the heat to a gentle simmer, cover, and cook for 15–20 minutes or until the water has been absorbed and the quinoa is tender. Set aside, keeping the lid on.

2 Heat the olive oil in a frying pan on medium heat, then add the zucchini and some salt and pepper. Cook for 1 minute on each side, then add the red onion, half of the lemon zest, the garlic, and the paprika. Cook for 1–2 more minutes, then add the mixture to the quinoa. Taste, season as needed, and set aside.

3 Mix the feta, cantaloupe, and the remaining lemon zest in a bowl. Set aside.

4 Make the dressing by mixing the extra virgin olive oil, apple cider vinegar, and Dijon mustard in a bowl, then season with salt and pepper to taste. Toss the dressing with the sugar snap peas and black sesame seeds. Set aside.

5 Spoon the quinoa into a serving bowl, then add the sugar snap peas mixture, feta mixture, and arugula. Sprinkle with the basil leaves (if using) and add the lemon wedge (if using).

the BUILD

 Start with quinoa

 Add in sugar snap peas, feta mixture, and arugula

 Finish with green and purple basil leaves and lemon wedge

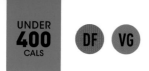

UNDER **400** CALS DF VG

Red rice & quinoa
with mango & mushrooms

prep **10 MIN**   cook **30 MIN**

Mushrooms and red rice give this bowl a nutty, earthy flavor that cuts through the tang of the herbs and mango.

Calories **344**	Cholesterol **0mg**	Dietary fiber **8.5g**
Total fat **4g**	Sodium **232mg**	Sugars **14g**
Saturated fat **0.5g**	Carbohydrates **59g**	Protein **13g**

the INGREDIENTS

½ cup quinoa

sea salt and freshly ground black pepper

1 tsp rice vinegar

½ cup red rice

1 tsp olive oil

1 cup button mushrooms, quartered

2 green onions, green part only from 1 and both finely chopped

½ garlic clove, finely chopped

1 tsp barley miso

¼ red onion, finely sliced

1 cup mango, cubed

handful of cilantro leaves, finely chopped

handful of spinach leaves

¼ red chili pepper, finely chopped

lime wedge (optional)

the PREP

1 Put the quinoa and a pinch of sea salt in a saucepan with 1 cup of water. Bring to a boil, then reduce the heat to a simmer, cover, and cook for 15–20 minutes. Let cool for 5 minutes, then stir in the rice vinegar.

2 Meanwhile, put the red rice, 1 cup of water, and a pinch of sea salt in a separate saucepan. Bring to a boil, then reduce the heat to a simmer, cover, and cook for 30 minutes (or according to the package instructions). Set aside, keeping the lid on.

3 Heat the olive oil in a nonstick frying pan over medium heat, and add the mushrooms, the green part from 1 green onion, and the garlic. Cook for 1–2 minutes, then add the miso and 2 tsp of water, cook for 2–3 more minutes, and set aside.

4 Stir the red onion, mango, cilantro leaves, and some salt and pepper into the red rice.

5 Spoon the red rice mixture into a serving bowl, then add the quinoa, mushrooms, and spinach leaves. Sprinkle the red chili pepper and the green and white parts from the remaining green onion and add the lime wedge (if using).

the BUILD

 Start with
red rice mixture

 Add in
quinoa, mushrooms, and spinach leaves

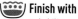 **Finish with**
red chili pepper, green onion, and lime wedge

UNDER 600 CALS

Quinoa & chickpeas
with lemon & tofu dressing

prep **10 MIN**   cook **25 MIN**

Chickpeas contain plenty of dietary fiber, but you'll also appreciate the zing from the lemon and tofu dressing.

Calories **590**	Cholesterol **0mg**	Dietary fiber **17.5g**
Total fat **22g**	Sodium **92mg**	Sugars **9g**
Saturated fat **3g**	Carbohydrates **54g**	Protein **35.5g**

the INGREDIENTS

½ cup white, black, and red quinoa mix

sea salt and freshly ground black pepper

1 tsp olive oil

½ cup firm tofu, cubed

½ cup frozen edamame, defrosted

½ cup cooked chickpeas

handful of flat-leaf parsley, finely chopped

½ red chili pepper, finely chopped

finely grated zest and juice of ½ lemon

handful of watercress

1 carrot, peeled into ribbons with a vegetable peeler

pinch of black sesame seeds

For the dressing

juice of 1 lemon

¼ cup silken tofu

1 tsp extra virgin olive oil

the PREP

1 Put the quinoa and a pinch of sea salt in a saucepan with 1 cup of water. Bring to a boil, then reduce the heat to a simmer, cover, and cook for 15–20 minutes or until tender. Set aside, keeping the lid on.

2 Heat the olive oil in a nonstick wok or frying pan over medium heat, then add the tofu. Cook for 5 minutes, stirring, until golden brown. Toss with the edamame, and set aside.

3 Mix the chickpeas, flat-leaf parsley, red chili pepper, and lemon zest and juice in a bowl, then season with salt and pepper. Set aside.

4 Make the dressing by blending the lemon juice, silken tofu, extra virgin olive oil, and some salt and pepper in a food processor. Set aside.

5 Spoon the quinoa into a serving bowl, then add the chickpea mixture, tofu mixture, watercress, and carrot. Drizzle the dressing and sprinkle the black sesame seeds.

the BUILD

 Start with
white, black, and red quinoa mixture

 Add in
chickpea mixture, edamame and tofu mixture, watercress, and carrot

 Finish with
lemon and tofu dressing and black sesame seeds

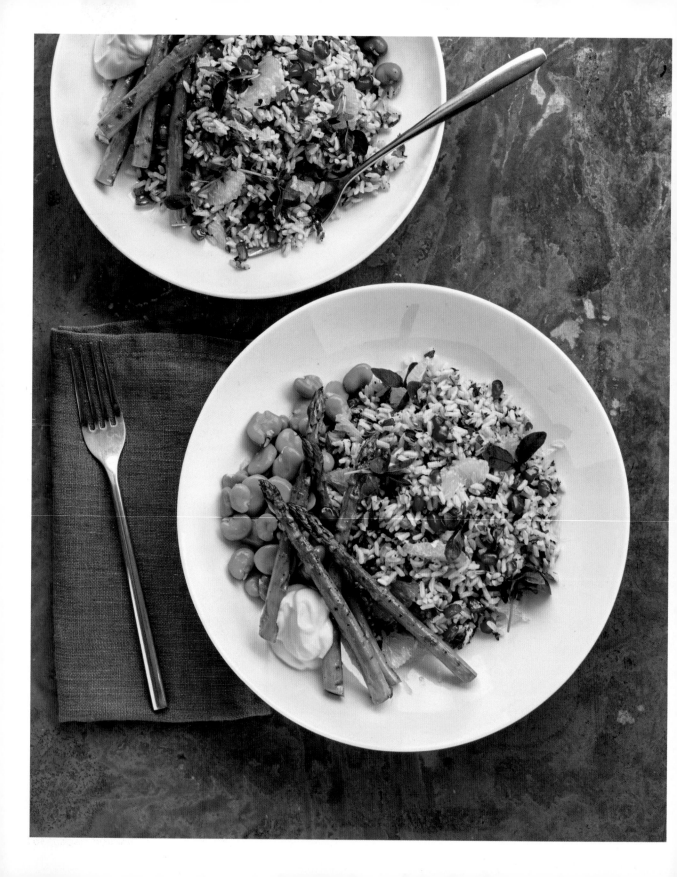

GF **UNDER 300 CALS**

Brown rice, cilantro & mint
with asparagus & fava beans

prep **15 MIN**   cook **40 MIN**

Brown rice makes a hearty base for the delicate green vegetables and fragrant herbs in this bowl.

Calories **290**	Cholesterol **0.1mg**	Dietary fiber **10g**
Total fat **6g**	Sodium **15mg**	Sugars **5g**
Saturated fat **1g**	Carbohydrates **42g**	Protein **12g**

the INGREDIENTS

1 cup brown rice

sea salt and freshly ground black pepper

5 asparagus spears

1 tsp olive oil

½ cup fava beans

handful of cilantro leaves, finely chopped, plus whole leaves (optional)

handful of mint leaves, finely chopped

1 lime, peeled, segmented, and halved

3 tsp pomegranate seeds

1 tsp 0% fat plain Greek yogurt

purple basil leaves (optional)

the PREP

1 Put the brown rice and some sea salt in a saucepan with 2¼ cups of water. Bring to a boil, then reduce the heat to a gentle simmer, cover, and cook for 25–30 minutes or until the water has been absorbed and the rice is tender. Set aside, keeping the lid on.

2 Meanwhile, put the asparagus in a bowl and toss with the olive oil and some salt and pepper. Heat a griddle pan over high heat, and cook the asparagus spears for 2–3 minutes on each side. Set aside.

3 Put the fava beans in a saucepan of boiling salted water, cook for 4 minutes or until tender, then drain, peel if desired, and set aside.

4 Mix the chopped cilantro leaves and mint leaves with the rice, season with salt and pepper, then add the lime segments and half the pomegranate seeds. Set aside.

5 Transfer the rice mixture to a serving bowl, then add the asparagus, fava beans, and the remaining pomegranate seeds. Spoon on the Greek yogurt, then sprinkle the whole cilantro leaves (if using) and basil leaves (if using).

the BUILD

 Start with
brown rice mixture

 Add in
asparagus, fava beans, and pomegranate seeds

 Finish with
yogurt, cilantro leaves, and basil leaves

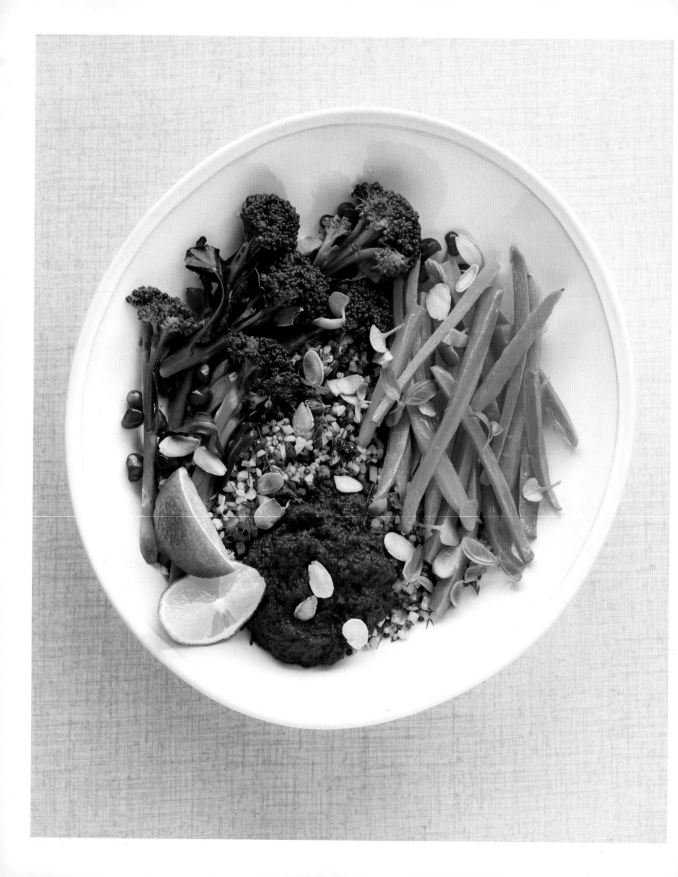

DF **VG**

UNDER
600
CALS

Bulgur wheat & roasted carrots
with beet-almond pesto

prep **20 MIN**   cook **35 MIN**

Beet-almond pesto is a delicious addition to this dish, a meal already boasting carrot "fries" and bulgur wheat.

Calories **520**	Cholesterol **0mg**	Dietary fiber **11g**
Total fat **13.5g**	Sodium **124mg**	Sugars **15g**
Saturated fat **1.5g**	Carbohydrates **76g**	Protein **18g**

the INGREDIENTS

2 carrots, peeled and cut into strips

1 tsp olive oil

sea salt and freshly ground black pepper

½ cup bulgur wheat and white and red quinoa mix, or other grain mix

¼ red onion, finely chopped

handful of chives, finely chopped

handful of dill, finely chopped

1 cup broccolini or regular broccoli florets, trimmed

2 tsp pomegranate seeds

1 tsp almond flakes, toasted (see p129)

handful of basil leaves (optional)

lime wedge (optional)

For the pesto

½ cup cooked beets

2 tsp almond flakes

handful of basil leaves

1 tsp extra virgin olive oil

pinch of red pepper flakes

the PREP

1 Preheat the oven to 400°F (200°C). Mix the carrots, olive oil, and some salt and pepper in a roasting pan. Roast for 20 minutes or until tender. Set aside.

2 Meanwhile, add the bulgur wheat and quinoa mix and some sea salt to a saucepan with 1 cup of water. Bring to a boil, then reduce the heat to a gentle simmer, cover, and cook for 15 minutes or until tender. Set aside, leaving the lid on, for 2–3 minutes, then stir in the red onion, chives, and dill. Set aside.

3 While the bulgur wheat cooks, steam the broccolini for 5–6 minutes or until tender. Set aside.

4 Make the pesto by blending the beets, almond flakes, basil leaves, extra virgin olive oil, red pepper flakes, and some salt and pepper in a food processor. Set aside.

5 Transfer the bulgur and quinoa mix to a serving bowl, then add the carrots, broccolini, and pomegranate seeds. Spoon on the beet-almond pesto, sprinkle with the toasted almond flakes and basil leaves (if using), then add the lime wedge (if using).

the BUILD

 Start with
bulgur and quinoa mixture

 Add in
carrots, broccolini, and pomegranate seeds

Finish with
pesto, almond flakes, basil leaves, and lime wedge

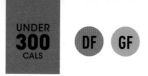

UNDER **300** CALS DF GF

Poached lemongrass chicken
with shiitake mushrooms

prep **15 MIN**   cook **25 MIN**

Poaching is a healthy cooking method that produces tender, juicy meat—great paired with earthy veggies and bright herbs.

Calories **295**	Cholesterol **87mg**	Dietary fiber **4g**
Total fat **12g**	Sodium **137mg**	Sugars **6g**
Saturated fat **7g**	Carbohydrates **8g**	Protein **35g**

the INGREDIENTS

4½ oz (125g) skinless chicken breast

sea salt and freshly ground black pepper

½ cup reduced-fat coconut milk

½ stalk of lemongrass, trimmed and outer layer removed

1 bay leaf (optional)

1 cup bok choy, trimmed and leaves separated

1 tsp sesame seeds

3 shiitake mushrooms

handful of cilantro leaves, half chopped

lime wedges (optional)

For the dressing

1 tsp mirin rice wine

½ tsp honey

½ tsp red chili pepper, finely chopped

the PREP

1 Place the chicken breast in a saucepan and season with salt and pepper. Pour in the coconut milk and ½ cup of water, then add the lemongrass and bay leaf (if using). Bring to just below a boil, then reduce the heat to a gentle simmer. Cover and cook for 15 minutes or until the juices from the chicken run clear when the chicken is pierced with a sharp knife. Remove the chicken from the liquid with a slotted spoon, set aside, and discard the liquid and aromatics.

2 While the chicken cooks, make the dressing by mixing the mirin, honey, red chili pepper, and some salt in a bowl. Set aside.

3 Steam the bok choy for 3 minutes or until tender. Set aside.

4 Place the sesame seeds in a small frying pan over medium-low heat and cook, stirring, until they turn a shade darker and smell toasted. Transfer to a plate and set aside.

5 Place the shiitake mushrooms in a nonstick frying pan over high heat and cook for 3–4 minutes or until tender. Set aside.

6 Slice the chicken and put it in a serving bowl, then add the bok choy and mushrooms. Scatter the chopped and whole cilantro leaves, spoon on the dressing, sprinkle the sesame seeds, and add the lime wedges (if using).

the BUILD

 Start with
chicken, bok choy, and mushrooms

 Add in
cilantro leaves and mirin dressing

 Finish with
sesame seeds and lime wedges

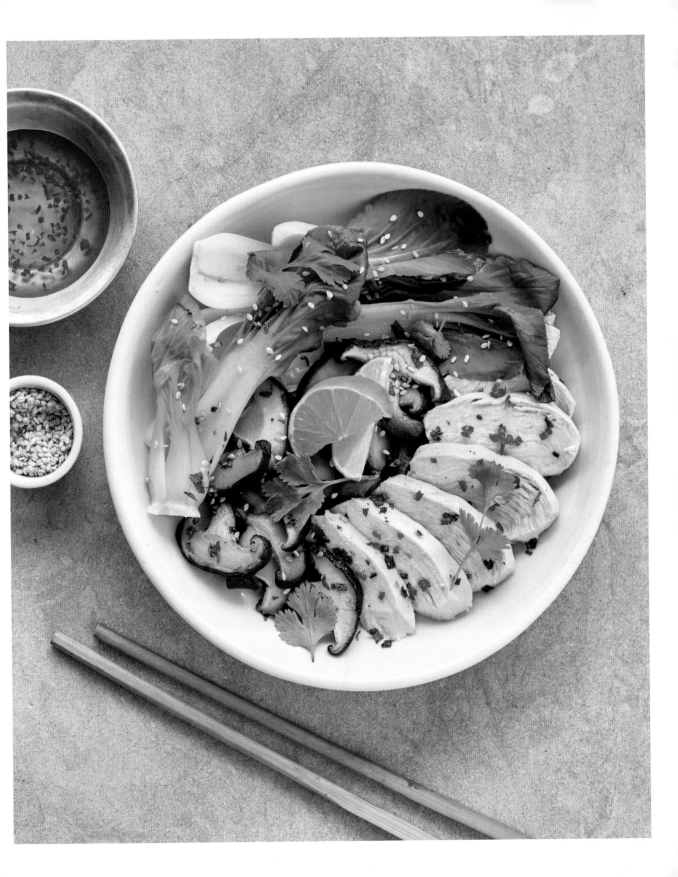

Brown rice & sweet potato
with kidney bean salsa

prep **10 MIN**   cook **45 MIN**

This bowl offers healthy Tex-Mex flavors: smoky paprika, cooling yogurt, and creamy avocado.

Calories **598**	Cholesterol **0mg**	Dietary fiber **17.5g**
Total fat **16g**	Sodium **53mg**	Sugars **12.5g**
Saturated fat **3g**	Carbohydrates **89g**	Protein **16g**

the INGREDIENTS

½ cup brown rice, rinsed and drained

sea salt and freshly ground black pepper

1 sweet potato, peeled and cut into chunky pieces

1 tsp olive oil

pinch of ground cinnamon

½ cup red kidney beans

handful of cilantro leaves, finely chopped, plus a few leaves for garnish

1 tbsp 0% fat plain Greek yogurt

juice of ½ lime

½ small avocado

juice of 1 lemon

For the salsa

2 tomatoes

1 green onion, roughly chopped

½ red chili pepper, roughly chopped

½ tsp smoked or regular paprika

the PREP

1 Preheat the oven to 400°F (200°C). Add the rice to a saucepan. Pour in 1½ cups of water and add a pinch of sea salt. Bring to a boil, then reduce the heat to a gentle simmer, cover, and cook for 30 minutes or until the water has been absorbed and the rice is tender. Set aside, keeping the lid on.

2 Mix the sweet potato, olive oil, cinnamon, and some salt and pepper in a roasting pan. Roast for 15 minutes or until the potatoes are tender and a pale golden brown. Set aside.

3 Make the salsa by blending the tomatoes, green onion, red chili pepper, and paprika in a food processor. Pour the salsa into a bowl and stir in the red kidney beans, half of the chopped cilantro, and some salt and pepper. Set aside.

4 Mix the Greek yogurt, lime juice, and the remaining chopped cilantro leaves in a bowl. Chop the avocado and toss it in the lemon juice to prevent discoloration.

5 Spoon the brown rice into a serving bowl, then add the salsa, sweet potato, and avocado. Spoon on the yogurt mix, then sprinkle the whole cilantro leaves.

the BUILD

 Start with
brown rice

 Add in
tomato and kidney bean salsa, sweet potato, and avocado

 Finish with
yogurt mixture and cilantro leaves

Bulgur wheat & chickpeas
with lemon & mint dressing

prep **15 MIN**   cook **20 MIN**

Roasting vegetables intensifies their sweetness and makes them great additions to nutty bulgur wheat.

Calories **500**	Cholesterol **0mg**	Dietary fiber **17g**
Total fat **11g**	Sodium **38mg**	Sugars **13g**
Saturated fat **1.6g**	Carbohydrates **72g**	Protein **19g**

the INGREDIENTS

1 carrot, peeled and roughly chopped

1 cup butternut squash, peeled and roughly chopped

1 tsp olive oil

pinch of zatar

sea salt and freshly ground black pepper

6 cherry tomatoes

⅓ cup bulgur wheat

½ cup cooked chickpeas

1 cup raw spinach leaves

1 tsp roughly chopped pistachios

For the dressing

1 tsp olive oil

1 tsp white wine vinegar

juice of ½ lemon

¼ tsp honey

handful of mint leaves, finely chopped

the PREP

1 Preheat the oven to 400°F (200°C). Mix the carrot, squash, olive oil, zatar, and some salt and pepper in a roasting pan. Roast for 15–20 minutes or until tender. Add the cherry tomatoes for the last 10 minutes, remove the pan from the oven, and set aside.

2 While the vegetables roast, put the bulgur wheat and some sea salt in a saucepan with ⅔ cup of water. Bring to a boil, then reduce the heat to a simmer, cover, and cook for 10–15 minutes or until the bulgur wheat is tender and the water has been absorbed. Set aside, keeping the lid on.

3 Make the dressing by whisking the olive oil, white wine vinegar, lemon juice, honey, mint leaves, and some salt and pepper in a bowl. Set aside.

4 Add the carrot, squash, tomatoes, and half the dressing to the bulgur wheat, toss well, and set aside.

5 Mix the remaining dressing with the chickpeas. Set aside.

6 Spoon the bulgur wheat mixture and the chickpeas into a serving bowl, then add the spinach leaves and sprinkle the pistachios.

the BUILD

 Start with
bulgur wheat mixture and chickpeas

 Add in
spinach leaves

 Finish with
pistachios

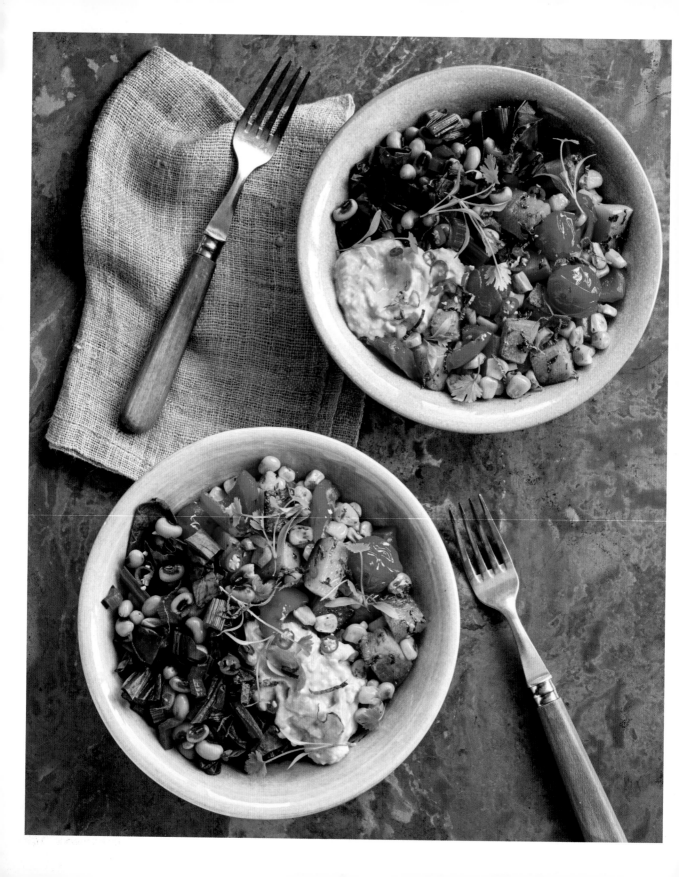

Black-eyed peas & squash
with avocado dressing

prep **15 MIN**   cook **20 MIN**

This creamy avocado dressing pairs beautifully with a spicy roasted vegetables and bean mixture.

Calories **470**	Cholesterol **0mg**	Dietary fiber **15.5g**
Total fat **27g**	Sodium **226mg**	Sugars **11g**
Saturated fat **5g**	Carbohydrates **34g**	Protein **15.5g**

the INGREDIENTS

½ cup butternut squash, peeled

pinch of ground cinnamon

2 tsp olive oil

sea salt and freshly ground black pepper

¼ red bell pepper, roughly chopped

5 cherry tomatoes

pinch of dried oregano

½ cup sweet corn

¼ tsp white wine vinegar

handful of mint leaves, chopped

6 stems of red or regular chard

½ cup cooked black-eyed peas

¼ red chili pepper, sliced

a few herbs, such as cilantro leaves (optional)

For the dressing

½ avocado

1 tbsp 0% fat plain Greek yogurt

1 tsp extra virgin olive oil

juice of ¼ lemon

the PREP

1 Preheat the oven to 400°F (200°C). Mix the squash, cinnamon, 1 tsp of the olive oil, and some salt and pepper in a roasting pan. Toss the red bell pepper with a drizzle of olive oil before adding it to the pan, then roast the vegetables for 15–20 minutes. Set aside.

2 Toss the cherry tomatoes, oregano, and a drizzle of olive oil in a bowl, then add the tomatoes and sweet corn to the roasting pan for the last 10 minutes of cooking. Remove the pan from the oven, transfer the tomatoes and corn to a bowl, mix in the white wine vinegar and mint leaves, and set aside.

3 While the tomatoes and sweet corn roast, steam the chard for 4 minutes or until tender. When the chard is cooled, roughly chop it, toss it with warmed black-eyed peas, and set aside.

4 Make the dressing by mashing together the avocado, Greek yogurt, extra virgin olive oil, lemon juice, and some salt and pepper in a bowl until smooth. Set aside.

5 Spoon the bean mixture into a serving bowl, then add the roasted vegetables. Spoon on the dressing and scatter the red chili pepper slices and the herbs (if using).

the BUILD

 Start with
black-eyed peas

 Add in
butternut squash, tomatoes, sweet corn, and red bell pepper

Finish with
red chili pepper, mint leaves, avocado dressing, and herbs

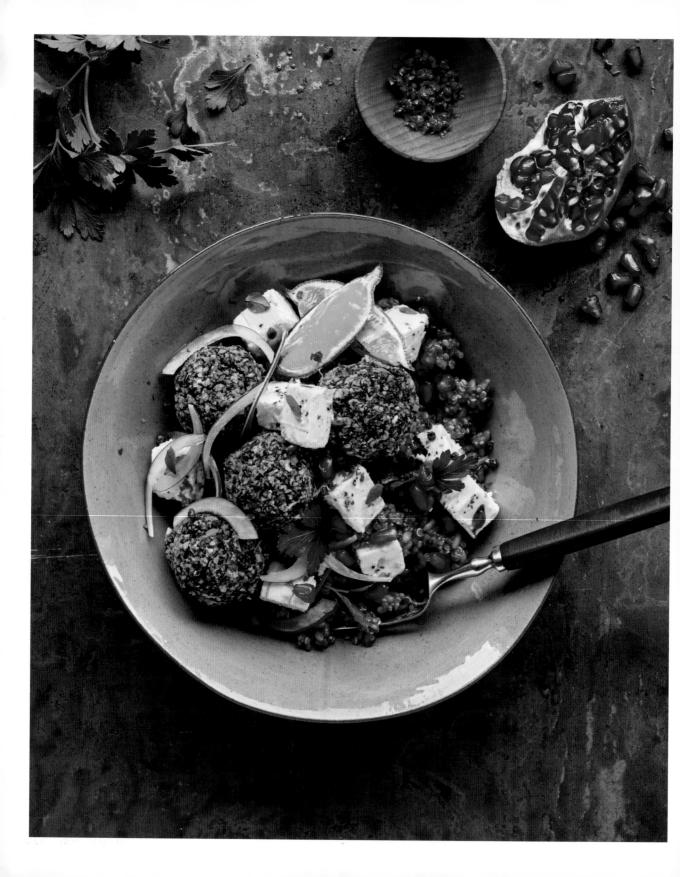

UNDER
600
CALS

Spiced freekeh
with chickpea & spinach balls

prep **20 MIN**   cook **15 MIN**

This makes a double portion of the balls, allowing you to save some prep—and have another great meal another day.

Calories **582**	Cholesterol **14mg**	Dietary fiber **25g**
Total fat **14.5g**	Sodium **1,204mg**	Sugars **9g**
Saturated fat **4g**	Carbohydrates **72g**	Protein **28g**

the INGREDIENTS

½ cup quick-cook freekeh and quinoa mix

⅓ cup tomato purée

pinch of sumac

pinch of red pepper flakes

¼ cup feta cheese, cubed

finely grated zest of ¼ lemon

a few thyme leaves

¼ red onion, finely chopped

1 tsp pomegranate seeds

½ tsp pink peppercorns, crushed

a few flat-leaf parsley leaves (optional)

For the balls

1 cup spinach leaves

1 cup cooked chickpeas

pinch of ground cumin

pinch of sumac

sea salt and freshly ground black pepper

lemon wedges

the PREP

1   Preheat the oven to 400°F (200°C). Steam the spinach until it wilts, then drain, pressing it in a sieve to remove all the excess water. Blend the chickpeas in a food processor until they're well chopped but retain some texture. Add the spinach, cumin, sumac, and some salt and pepper, then blend again using the pulse button until the mixture comes together. Form the mixture into 8 balls and place them on a nonstick baking sheet, along with the lemon wedges. Bake for 15 minutes or until the balls start to turn a pale golden brown. Set aside.

2   While the balls bake, put the freekeh and quinoa mix in a saucepan, add the tomato purée, just cover with water, and add a pinch of sea salt. Bring to a boil, then reduce the heat to a simmer, cover, and cook for 10 minutes or until tender. Remove from the heat, then stir in the sumac, red pepper flakes, and some salt and pepper. Set aside.

3   Toss the feta, zest, thyme, and onion in a bowl. Set aside.

4   Put the freekeh mixture in a serving bowl, then arrange 4 balls and the lemon wedges on top. Spoon in the feta mixture and scatter the pomegranate seeds, pink peppercorns, and parsley (if using). (Refrigerate the remaining balls in an airtight container and use them within 2 days.)

the BUILD

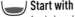 **Start with**
freekeh and quinoa mixture

 Add in
chickpea balls, lemon wedges, and feta mixture

Finish with
pomegranate seeds, pink peppercorns, and flat-leaf parsley

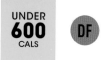

UNDER **600** CALS · DF

Korean beef & rice
with pickled red cabbage

prep **20 MIN**   cook **20 MIN**

Diverse colors and textures surround flavorful beef and red cabbage in this feast for the eyes—and the appetite.

Calories **562**	Cholesterol **64mg**	Dietary fiber **11.5g**
Total fat **18g**	Sodium **887mg**	Sugars **11g**
Saturated fat **4g**	Carbohydrates **53g**	Protein **41.5g**

the INGREDIENTS

4½ oz (125g) sirloin steak, fat removed

2 tsp rice vinegar

pinch of red pepper flakes

¼ tsp honey

1 cup red cabbage, shredded

4 stalks broccolini, trimmed

½ cup carrot, sliced into strips

8 stalks of red or regular chard, trimmed

1 cup cooked quinoa and whole-grain rice mix, cooked

pinch of black sesame seeds

a few cilantro leaves (optional)

lime wedges (optional)

For the marinade

1 tsp sesame oil

2 tsp dark soy sauce

1 tsp rice vinegar

¼ tsp peeled and grated fresh ginger

¼ tsp peeled and grated garlic

juice of ¼ lime

pinch of red pepper flakes

sea salt and freshly ground black pepper

the PREP

1 Make the marinade by mixing the sesame oil, dark soy sauce, rice vinegar, ginger, garlic, lime juice, red pepper flakes, and some salt and pepper in a bowl. Add the steak to the bowl and marinate for 10 minutes.

2 While the steak marinates, mix the rice vinegar, red pepper flakes, and honey in a bowl, then add the red cabbage. Season with some salt and pepper, toss, and set aside.

3 Heat a griddle pan over high heat and add the steak and marinade. Cook on both sides until done to your liking, then allow to rest for 5–10 minutes. Slice into strips and set aside.

4 Steam the broccolini for 2 minutes, then add the carrot and steam for 2 more minutes. Add the chard and steam for another 1–2 minutes or until all the vegetables are tender but still retain a bite to them. Set aside.

5 Spoon the quinoa and whole-grain rice mix into a serving bowl, then add the steak, steamed vegetables, and red cabbage. Sprinkle the black sesame seeds, scatter the cilantro leaves (if using), and add the lime wedges (if using).

the BUILD

 Start with
quinoa and whole-grain rice mix

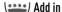 **Add in**
steak, steamed vegetables, and red cabbage

 Finish with
black sesame seeds, cilantro leaves, and lime wedges

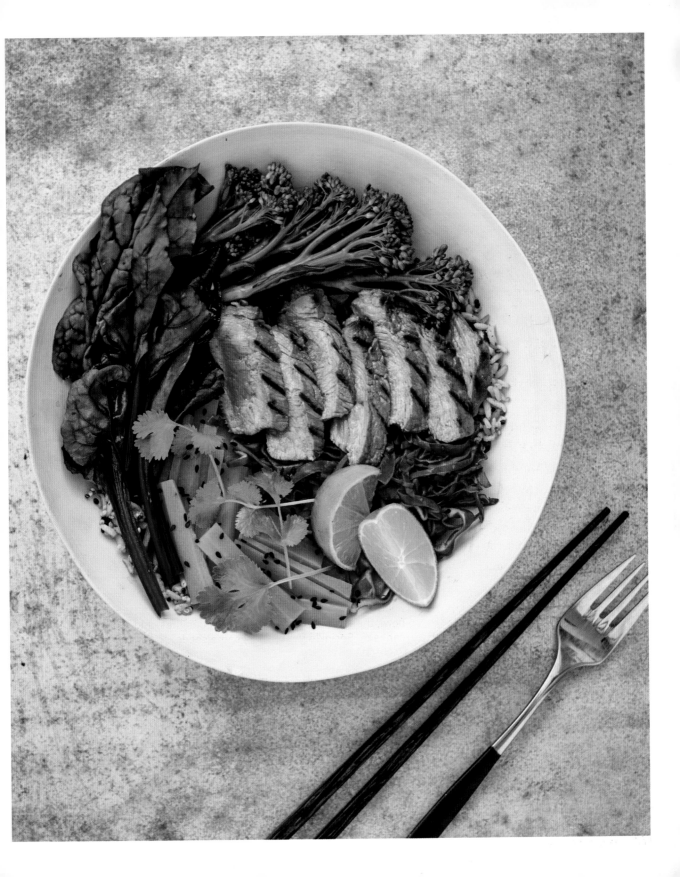

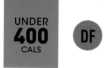

UNDER 400 CALS **DF**

Turkey meatballs & noodles
with tahini & honey dressing

prep **15 MIN**   cook **35 MIN**

Turkey is a fantastic low-fat protein. For this bowl, it's mixed with fresh herbs and a nutty tahini dressing.

Calories **364**	Cholesterol **57g**	Dietary fiber **4g**
Total fat **11.5g**	Sodium **107g**	Sugars **5g**
Saturated fat **2g**	Carbohydrates **32g**	Protein **32g**

the INGREDIENTS

3½ oz (100g) turkey steak

finely grated zest of ½ lemon

handful of flat-leaf parsley

pinch of sumac

sea salt and freshly ground black pepper

1 tsp olive oil

7 cherry tomatoes

1½ oz (40g) soba noodles

2 cups kale, coarse stalks removed and leaves roughly chopped

lemon wedge (optional)

For the dressing

1 tsp olive oil

1 tsp white wine vinegar

1 tsp tahini

¼ tsp honey

the PREP

1 Preheat the oven to 400°F (200°C). Blend the turkey, lemon zest, flat-leaf parsley, sumac, and some salt and pepper in a food processor. Brush a roasting pan with ½ tsp of the olive oil, form the mixture into 4 balls, and place them in the pan. Bake for 20 minutes, turning halfway, and set aside.

2 Mix the cherry tomatoes, the remaining olive oil, and some salt and pepper in a separate roasting pan. Roast for 10–15 minutes or until lightly charred and the skins begin to burst. Set aside.

3 Put the soba noodles in a bowl and cover with boiling water. Leave for 5–10 minutes (or according to package instructions), drain, then rinse with cold water to separate. Set aside.

4 Steam the kale for 10 minutes or until tender. Set aside.

5 Make the tahini and honey dressing by whisking the olive oil, white wine vinegar, tahini, honey, and some salt and pepper in a bowl. Set aside.

6 Transfer the soba noodles to a serving bowl, then add the turkey balls, kale, tomatoes, and lemon wedge (if using) to squeeze over. Drizzle the tahini and honey dressing.

the BUILD

 Start with
soba noodles

 Add in
turkey balls, kale, tomatoes, and lemon wedge

 Finish with
tahini and honey dressing

DF

UNDER 400 CALS

Soba noodles & kale
with sesame seed dressing

prep 15 MIN   cook 20 MIN

This is a colorful bowl of tasty and nutritional goodness—kale is full of iron and the egg is rich in protein.

Calories **390**	Cholesterol **213mg**	Dietary fiber **6g**
Total fat **12g**	Sodium **439mg**	Sugars **7g**
Saturated fat **3g**	Carbohydrates **46g**	Protein **21g**

the INGREDIENTS

1 cup kale, coarse stalks removed and leaves roughly chopped

1 egg

2 oz (60g) soba noodles

½ cup red cabbage, shredded

1 tsp rice vinegar

½ cup frozen edamame, defrosted

½ sheet nori, finely chopped

pinch of black sesame seeds

a few cilantro leaves

For the dressing

1 tsp extra virgin olive oil

1 tsp white wine vinegar

1 tsp sesame seeds

¼ tsp honey (optional)

sea salt and freshly ground black pepper

the PREP

1 Steam the kale for 10 minutes or until tender. Set aside.

2 While the kale steams, make the dressing by whisking the extra virgin olive oil, white wine vinegar, sesame seeds, honey (if using), and some salt and pepper in a bowl. Set aside.

3 Put the egg into a saucepan with enough cold water to cover, bring to a boil, and cook for 5 minutes, then drain and plunge into cold water. Once the egg is cool enough to handle, peel and halve it. Set aside.

4 Put the soba noodles in a bowl and cover with boiling water. Leave for 5 minutes (or according to the package instructions), drain, rinse with cold water to separate, and set aside.

5 Toss the red cabbage and rice vinegar in a bowl. Set aside.

6 Transfer the soba noodles to a serving bowl, then add the kale, red cabbage mixture, edamame, nori, and egg halves. Sprinkle the sesame seeds, drizzle the sesame seed dressing, and scatter the cilantro leaves.

the BUILD

 Start with soba noodles

 Add in kale, red cabbage mixture, edamame, and egg

 Finish with sesame seeds, sesame seed dressing, and cilantro leaves

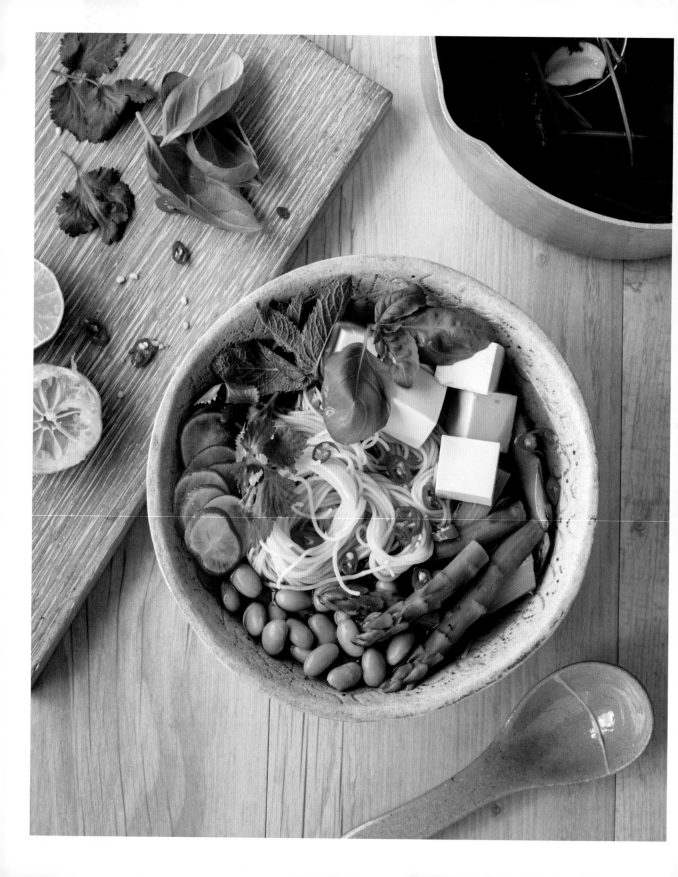

Spring vegetable pho
with vermicelli noodles

prep **15 MIN**   cook **30 MIN**

A great pick-me-up soup you can enjoy all year; just adjust the vegetables according to what's in season.

Calories **172**	Cholesterol **0mg**	Dietary fiber **3.5g**
Total fat **3.5g**	Sodium **557mg**	Sugars **3.5g**
Saturated fat **0.5g**	Carbohydrates **24g**	Protein **10.5g**

the INGREDIENTS

1 cup vermicelli rice noodles

5 asparagus spears, halved

⅓ cup frozen edamame beans, defrosted

⅓ cup firm tofu, cut into cubes

For the broth

½ cinnamon stick

1 star anise

1-in (2.5cm) piece of fresh ginger, peeled and chopped

½ garlic clove

2 tsp dark soy sauce, or to taste

2 tsp rice vinegar, or to taste

handful of cilantro stalks

sea salt and freshly ground black pepper

For the topping

1 radish, finely sliced

a few Thai basil leaves

a few mint leaves

a few cilantro leaves

½ red chili pepper, finely sliced

lime wedge (optional)

the PREP

1 Put the vermicelli noodles in a bowl and cover them with boiling water for 10 minutes, then drain, and set aside.

2 Make the broth by putting the cinnamon stick, star anise, ginger, garlic, dark soy sauce, rice vinegar, and cilantro stalks in a saucepan with 2½ cups of water. Bring to a boil, then reduce the heat to a gentle simmer, cover, and cook for about 20 minutes. Drain through a colander, catching the clear broth in a clean saucepan, and season with salt and pepper. Taste, and add a little more soy sauce or rice vinegar if desired.

3 Put the broth back over medium heat and bring to a gentle simmer. Add the asparagus and edamame and cook for 5 minutes, or until the asparagus is just tender but still retains some bite. Add the tofu and simmer gently for 2 more minutes.

4 Transfer the vermicelli noodles to a serving bowl, then ladle the ginger broth and vegetables over the noodles. Scatter with the radish, Thai basil leaves, mint leaves, and cilantro leaves. Sprinkle with the red chili pepper, and add the lime wedge (if using), to squeeze over.

the BUILD

 Start with vermicelli noodles, ginger broth, and vegetables

 Add in radish, Thai basil leaves, mint leaves, and cilantro leaves

 Finish with red chili pepper and lime wedge

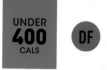

Saffron chicken
with lentils & orange

prep **15 MIN**   cook **30 MIN**

Saffron gives a subtle accent to roasted chicken, while green lentils tumbled with orange add some zing.

Calories **381**	Cholesterol **88mg**	Dietary fiber **9.5g**
Total fat **9.5g**	Sodium **389mg**	Sugars **18g**
Saturated fat **1.5g**	Carbohydrates **29g**	Protein **40g**

the INGREDIENTS

4½oz (125g) skinless chicken breast

2 tsp olive oil

pinch of saffron threads

sea salt and freshly ground black pepper

1 cup green beans, trimmed

1 tsp harissa

½ cup zucchini, sliced

1 cup cooked green lentils

1 orange, peeled and segmented

handful of mint leaves, finely chopped

handful of dill leaves, finely chopped

1 tomato, halved, seeds removed, and flesh finely chopped

a few mint leaves (optional)

lime wedge (optional)

the PREP

1 Preheat the oven to 400°F (200°C). Score the chicken breast a few times, and mix it with 1 tsp of the olive oil and the saffron in a roasting pan, then season with salt and pepper. Roast for 20 minutes, or until the juices run clear when the chicken is pierced with a sharp knife. Once the chicken is cool enough to handle, slice it on the diagonal.

2 Meanwhile, add the green beans to a pan of boiling water. Cook for 5 minutes, or until tender but still retaining some bite, then drain. Stir in the harissa and set aside.

3 Heat a griddle pan on high heat, then toss the zucchini with the remaining 1 tsp of olive oil in a bowl. Put the zucchini in the pan, cook for 2–3 minutes on each side or until golden brown, then remove from the pan.

4 Mix the green lentils, orange segments, mint leaves, and dill leaves in a bowl, seasoning with salt and pepper.

5 Transfer the green lentil mixture into a serving bowl, then add the saffron chicken, green beans, and zucchini. Spoon in the tomato, scatter with the mint leaves (if using), and add the lime wedge (if using) to squeeze over the bowl.

the BUILD

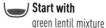 **Start with**
green lentil mixture

Add in
saffron chicken, green beans, and zucchini

 Finish with
tomatoes, mint leaves, and lime wedge

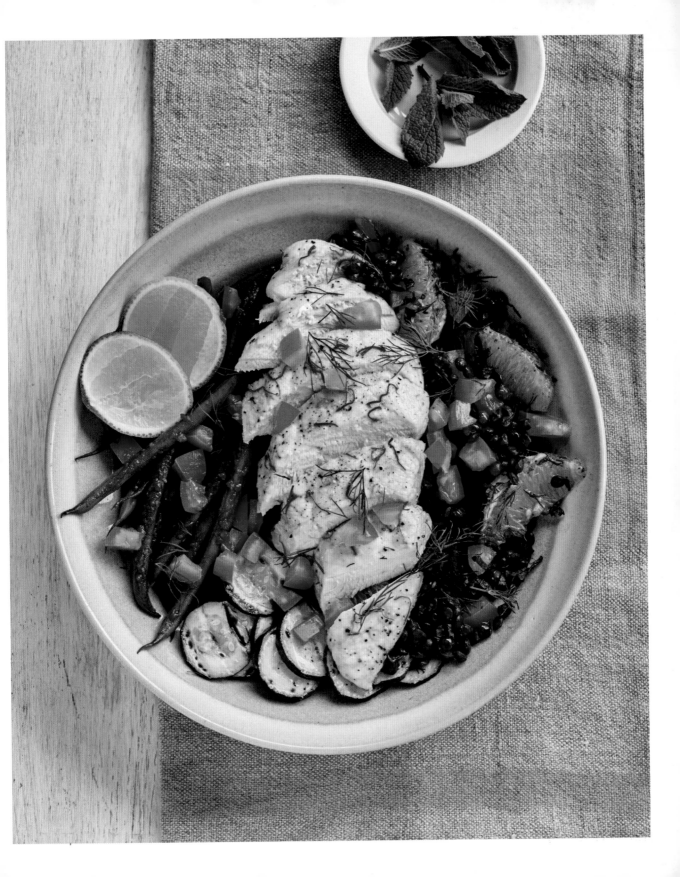

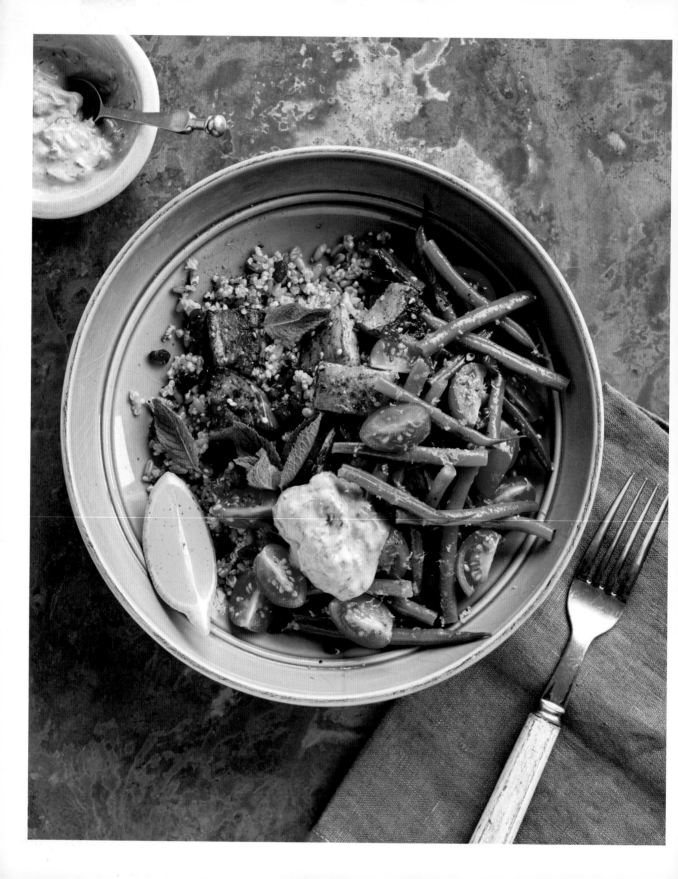

UNDER 400 CALS

Freekeh & eggplant
with harissa & mint dressing

prep **15 MIN**   cook **20 MIN**

This robust dish bursts with Middle Eastern flavors. The freekeh is a supergrain rich in protein and fiber.

Calories **315**	Cholesterol **0mg**	Dietary fiber **11g**
Total fat **5.5g**	Sodium **44mg**	Sugars **11g**
Saturated fat **1g**	Carbohydrates **48g**	Protein **13g**

the INGREDIENTS

½ cup freekeh and quinoa mix

sea salt and freshly ground black pepper

1 cup eggplant, roughly chopped

pinch of zatar

1 tsp olive oil

1 cup green beans, trimmed

finely grated zest of ½ lemon

5 cherry tomatoes, chopped

1 tsp barberries (soaked in water for 10 minutes)

sprig of mint leaves (optional)

lemon wedge (optional)

For the dressing

1 tbsp 0% fat plain Greek yogurt

1 tsp harissa

handful of mint leaves, finely chopped

the PREP

1 Put the freekeh and quinoa mix and some sea salt in a saucepan with 1 cup of water. Bring to a boil, then reduce the heat to a simmer, cover, and cook for 15 minutes (or according to the package instructions), or until tender. Remove from the heat, keeping the lid on.

2 Make the dressing by mixing the Greek yogurt, harissa, and mint leaves in a bowl, seasoning with salt and pepper. (This makes 2 portions. Store the extra portion in an airtight container in the fridge for up to 2 days.)

3 Toss the eggplant in a bowl with the zatar and olive oil, seasoning with salt and pepper. Heat a griddle pan on high heat, add the eggplant, cook for 2–3 minutes on each side or until golden brown, and set aside.

4 Meanwhile, add the green beans to a saucepan of boiling salted water. Cook for 5 minutes or until tender, drain, refresh with cold water, and drain again. Toss with the lemon zest and tomatoes.

5 Transfer the freekeh and quinoa mix to a serving bowl, then add the eggplant and green beans. Spoon in the yogurt dressing, scatter over the barberries and mint leaves (if using), and add the lemon wedge (if using).

the BUILD

 Start with
freekeh and quinoa mix

 Add in
eggplant, green beans, and yogurt dressing

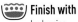 **Finish with**
barberries, mint leaves, and lemon wedge

UNDER 400 CALS **DF** **GF**

Peppered tuna & sweet potato
with cucumber-lemon relish

prep **10 MIN**   cook **25 MIN**

This is a colorful, crunchy bowl full of goodness, with a gentle kick from the tangy dressing.	Calories **381**	Cholesterol **248mg**	Dietary fiber **7g**
	Total fat **13g**	Sodium **216mg**	Sugars **10g**
	Saturated fat **3g**	Carbohydrates **25g**	Protein **37g**

the INGREDIENTS

1 sweet potato, peeled, and cut into chunky pieces

sea salt and freshly ground black pepper

1 egg

1 cup green beans

¼ cucumber, seeds removed, and sliced into half-moon shapes

6 radishes, finely sliced

1 lemon, peeled and segmented

handful of dill, chopped

3½ oz (100g) tuna steak

1 tsp olive oil

handful of flat-leaf parsley, finely chopped

For the dressing

1 tsp extra virgin olive oil

1 tsp white wine vinegar

1 tsp Dijon mustard

the PREP

1 Put the sweet potato in a saucepan with salted water to cover. Bring to a boil, reduce the heat to a simmer, cover, and cook for 10 minutes or until tender. Drain.

2 Put the egg into a saucepan with cold water to cover, bring to a boil, cook for 5 minutes, drain, then plunge into cold water. Once cool enough to handle, peel and halve it.

3 Meanwhile, make the dressing by whisking the extra virgin olive oil, white wine vinegar, and Dijon mustard in a bowl, seasoning with salt and pepper to taste.

4 Put the green beans in a saucepan of boiling salted water. Cook for 4 minutes or until tender, then drain.

5 Mix the cucumber, radishes, lemon segments, and dill, and season with salt and pepper.

6 Brush the tuna with the olive oil and season with pepper. Heat a griddle pan on high heat and cook for 3–4 minutes on each side, or until lightly charred. Cool a little, then slice.

7 Put the sweet potato in a serving bowl, then add the tuna, green beans, cucumber mixture, and egg. Drizzle with the dressing and scatter over the flat-leaf parsley.

the BUILD

 Start with
sweet potato

 Add in
tuna, green beans, cucumber mixture, and egg

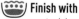 **Finish with**
mustard dressing and flat-leaf parsley

Roasted fennel & sea bass
with Dijon mustard dressing

prep **10 MIN**   cook **35 MIN**

A mix of flavors and textures, with delicious sea bass as a great source of protein and omega-3 fatty acids.

Calories **491**	Cholesterol **89mg**	Dietary fiber **8g**
Total fat **20g**	Sodium **98mg**	Sugars **9.5g**
Saturated fat **4g**	Carbohydrates **41g**	Protein **33g**

the INGREDIENTS

¼ fennel bulb, sliced lengthwise

½ red bell pepper, roughly chopped

½ red onion, half roughly chopped, half finely chopped

1 tsp olive oil

sea salt and freshly ground black pepper

4½ oz (125g) sea bass fillet, skinned

1 cup sugar snap peas, finely chopped

1 cup cooked brown rice

a few cilantro leaves (optional)

For the dressing

1 tsp extra virgin olive oil

1 tsp white wine vinegar

½ tsp Dijon mustard

the PREP

1 Preheat the oven to 400°F (200°C). Mix the fennel, red bell pepper, roughly chopped red onion, and olive oil in a roasting pan, then season with salt and pepper. Roast for 15–20 minutes.

2 Put the sea bass in another roasting pan, seasoning with salt and pepper, and pour in enough water to come one-third of the way up the pan. Cover with foil and roast for 10–15 minutes or until the fish is opaque and cooked. Remove the fish with a spatula and set aside.

3 Make the dressing by whisking the extra virgin olive oil, white wine vinegar, and Dijon mustard in a bowl, then season with salt and pepper to taste.

4 Mix the sugar snap peas, the finely chopped red onion, and half the dressing in a bowl.

5 Spoon the brown rice into a serving bowl, then add the sea bass and roasted vegetables. Sprinkle with the sugar snap peas mixture and cilantro leaves (if using), and drizzle with the remaining dressing.

the BUILD

 Start with
brown rice

 Add in
sea bass, vegetables, and sugar snap peas mixture

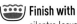 **Finish with**
cilantro leaves and mustard dressing

DF GF VG

Red rice & roasted squash
with mint dressing & almonds

prep **15 MIN**   cook **20 MIN**

Red rice has a nutty flavor that works well with the sweetness from the corn and butternut squash.

Calories **429**	Cholesterol **0mg**	Dietary fiber **8g**
Total fat **13.5g**	Sodium **22mg**	Sugars **8g**
Saturated fat **1.5g**	Carbohydrates **57g**	Protein **17g**

the INGREDIENTS

1 cup butternut squash, peeled, and cut into half-moon shapes

½ red bell pepper, roughly chopped

½ cup sweet corn

sea salt and freshly ground black pepper

1 tsp olive oil

½ cup red rice and wild rice mix

1 cup kale, coarse stalks removed, leaves roughly chopped

8 almonds, roughly chopped

For the dressing

2 tsp rice vinegar

handful of mint leaves, finely chopped

½ garlic clove, grated

the PREP

1 Preheat the oven to 400°F (200°C). Toss the squash in a roasting pan with the red bell pepper and sweet corn, seasoning with salt and pepper. Roast for 20 minutes or until tender.

2 Meanwhile, add the rice to a saucepan with sea salt and 1 cup of water. Bring to a boil, then reduce the heat to a gentle simmer, cover, and cook for 20 minutes or until the water has been absorbed and the rice is tender. Set aside, keeping the lid on.

3 Put the kale in a steamer, season with salt, then steam for 10 minutes or until tender.

4 Make the dressing by mixing the rice vinegar, mint leaves, and garlic in a bowl, seasoning with salt and pepper.

5 Spoon the rice mix into a serving bowl, then add the squash, red bell pepper, sweet corn, and kale. Sprinkle with the almonds and spoon the mint dressing over it.

the BUILD

 Start with
red rice and
wild rice mix

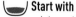 **Add in**
butternut squash,
red bell pepper,
sweet corn, and kale

 Finish with
almonds and
mint dressing

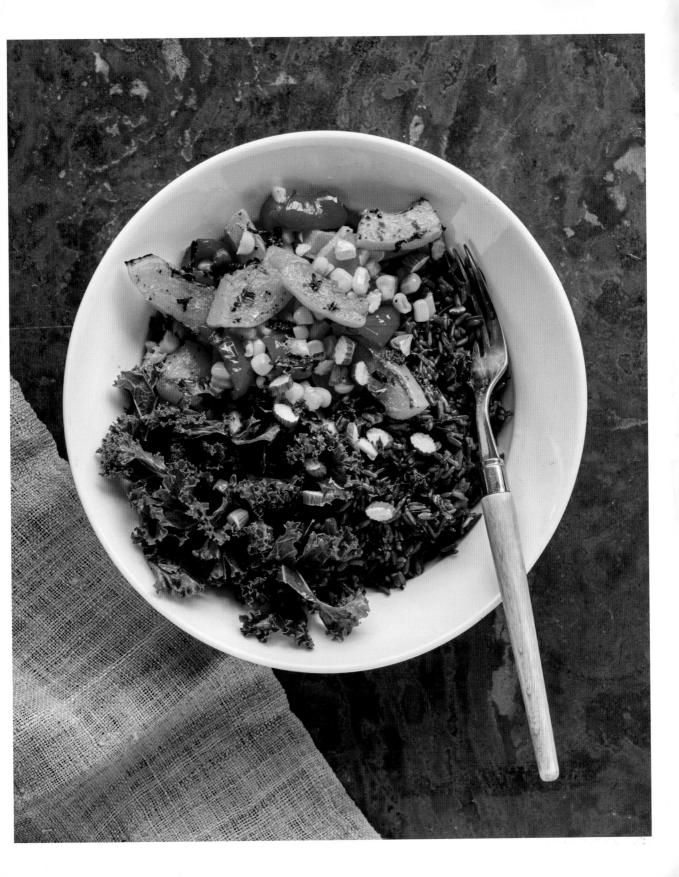

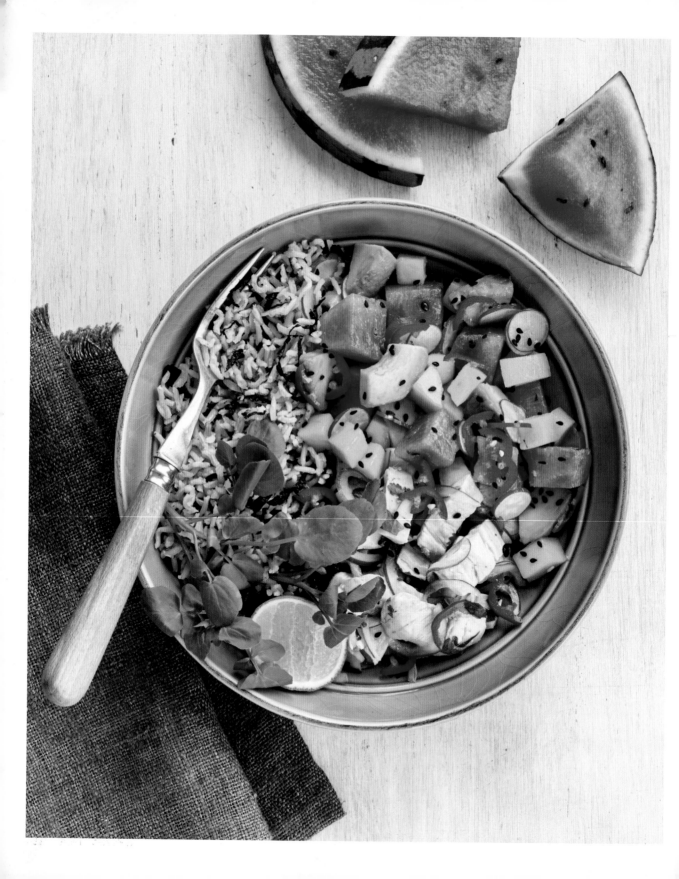

DF **GF**

UNDER 600 CALS

Brown rice & sea bass poke
with avocado & mango

prep **15 MIN**   cook **25 MIN**

Poke (pronounced *poh-kay*; it means "chunk" in Hawaiian) is a raw fish salad. It's colorful… and delicious.

Calories **598**	Cholesterol **71mg**	Dietary fiber **10g**
Total fat **28g**	Sodium **299mg**	Sugars **15g**
Saturated fat **6g**	Carbohydrates **54g**	Protein **29g**

the INGREDIENTS

½ cup brown rice

sea salt

4½ oz (125g) sea bass fillet, skinned and sliced with the grain into small, bite-sized pieces

½ red onion, finely sliced

juice of 1 lime, plus 1 lime wedge (optional)

handful of cilantro leaves, finely chopped

½ avocado

1 tsp rice vinegar

½ sheet nori, finely chopped

½ cup watermelon, cut into cubes

⅓ cup mango, cut into cubes

2 radishes, trimmed and finely sliced

handful of watercress

¼ red chili pepper, finely sliced

pinch of black sesame seeds

the PREP

1 Put the brown rice and some sea salt into a saucepan with 1 cup of water. Bring to a boil, then reduce the heat to a gentle simmer, cover, and cook for 20–25 minutes, or until the water has been absorbed and the rice is tender. Set aside, keeping the lid on.

2 Meanwhile, mix the sea bass, red onion, and a pinch of sea salt in a bowl. Let this sit for 1 minute before adding the juice of ½ lime and stirring again. Let it sit again for 5 minutes for the fish to "cook" in the citrus juice, then stir in the cilantro leaves. Chop the avocado into pieces roughly the same size as the mango and mix it with the juice of the remaining ½ lime to prevent discoloration.

3 Fluff the rice with a fork, then stir in the rice vinegar and dried nori.

4 Spoon the rice into a serving bowl and spoon the sea bass mixture over it, then add the watermelon, mango, avocado, radishes, and watercress. Sprinkle with the red chili pepper and black sesame seeds and add the lime wedge (if using), to squeeze over the bowl.

the BUILD

 Start with
brown rice
and sea bass mixture

 Add in
watermelon, mango,
avocado, radishes,
and watercress

 Finish with
red chili pepper, black
sesame seeds, and
lime wedge

Index

About the author

Heather Whinney is an experienced home economist, culinary writer, and food stylist. She has served as the food editor for several national magazines in the United Kingdom. She's the author of *Cook Express, Diabetes Cookbook*, and *The Gluten-Free Cookbook* (all by DK Books), and she was also the culinary school manager at Cordon Vert, where she developed her love of writing recipes.

Acknowledgments

Many thanks to Christopher Stolle, my development editor, and Brook Farling, my acquisitions editor, for all their guidance and patience along the way; William Thomas, for his fantastic designs; Fiona Hunter for her nutritional analysis; Trish Sebben-Krupka for her recipe testing; and to everyone involved with the photography for and production of this book. I couldn't have written this book without such a great team supporting me.

In fact, the whole process of developing and writing the recipes for this book has been a real pleasure. Bowl food has definitely become my number-one choice as a way of eating; for ease and taste and for the sheer comfort and satisfaction it gives, it has reinforced my love of healthy eating. I love punchy-flavored food, and the recipes in this book should reflect that. If you're embarking on a healthy eating regimen or weight loss plan, the last thing you need is bland food or you'll fall at the first hurdle. I hope you enjoy the flavor combinations in this book as much as I do.

Enjoy!

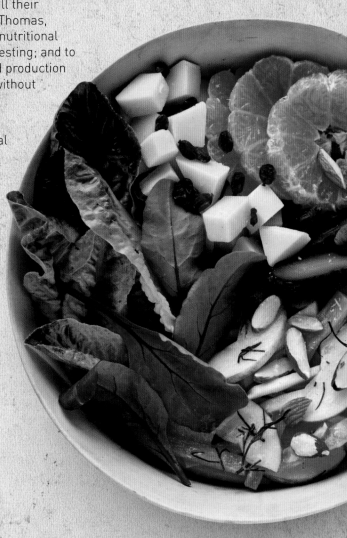

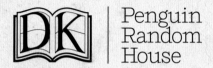

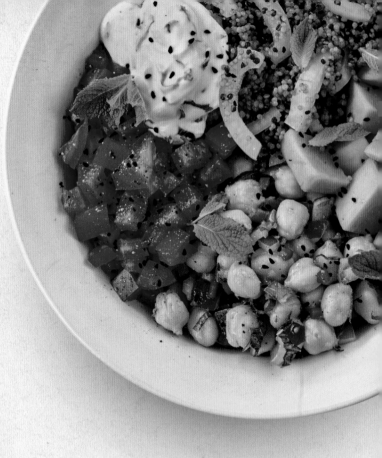

Acquisitions editor: Brook Farling
Development editor: Christopher Stolle
Book designer: William Thomas
Art directors: Maxine Pedliham, Christine Keilty, Glenda Fisher
Photographer: William Reavell
Food stylists: Maud Eden, Penny Stephens, and Kate Wesson
Prop stylist: Robert Merrett
Recipe reviewer: Trish Sebben-Krupka
Nutritional analysis: Fiona Hunter
Jacket designer: Steven Marsden
Prepress technician: Brian Massey
Proofreader: Amy Borrelli
Indexer: Celia McCoy
Associate publisher: Billy Fields
Publisher: Mike Sanders

First American Edition, 2017
Published in the United States by DK Publishing
6081 E. 82nd Street, Indianapolis, Indiana 46250

Copyright © 2017 Dorling Kindersley Limited
A Penguin Random House Company
17 18 19 20   10 9 8 7 6 5 4 3 2
002–304411–January/2017

All rights reserved.
Without limiting the rights under the copyright reserved above, no part of this publication may be reproduced, stored in or introduced into a retrieval system, or transmitted, in any form, or by any means (electronic, mechanical, photocopying, recording, or otherwise), without the prior written permission of the copyright owner.

Published in the United States by
Dorling Kindersley Limited.

ISBN: 978-1-4654-6159-9
Library of Congress Catalog Number: 2016947992

Printed and bound in China

All images © Dorling Kindersley Limited
For further information see: www.dkimages.com

A WORLD OF IDEAS:
SEE ALL THERE IS TO KNOW
www.dk.com

Note:
This publication contains the opinions and ideas of its author(s). It is intended to provide helpful and informative material on the subject matter covered. It is sold with the understanding that the author(s) and publisher are not engaged in rendering professional services in the book. If the reader requires personal assistance or advice, a competent professional should be consulted. The author(s) and publisher specifically disclaim any responsibility for any liability, loss, or risk, personal or otherwise, which is incurred as a consequence, directly or indirectly, of the use and application of any of the contents of this book.

Trademarks:
All terms mentioned in this book that are known to be or are suspected of being trademarks or service marks have been appropriately capitalized. Alpha Books, DK, and Penguin Random House LLC cannot attest to the accuracy of this information. Use of a term in this book should not be regarded as affecting the validity of any trademark or service mark.

DK books are available at special discounts when purchased in bulk for sales promotions, premiums, fund-raising, or educational use. For details, contact: DK Publishing Special Markets, 345 Hudson Street, New York, New York 10014 or SpecialSales@dk.com.